# Unlocking Herbal Antivirals

## A Comprehensive Guide to Natural Immune Boosters

# Helena Brooks

# Table of Contents

# INTRODUCTION

A Comprehensive Guide to Natural Immune Boosters" explores the field of herbal medicine and gives readers a thorough grasp of the immune-boosting potential of plant-based antivirals. Written by professionals in the field of herbal medicine, this book is an invaluable tool for anybody looking for non-traditional methods to improve their immunity to viral infections and overall well-being.

Readers will find a plethora of knowledge on several plants known for their antiviral qualities within their pages, including their historical use, scientific proof of their effectiveness, and proper preparation and administration techniques. Every herb, from well-known ones like licorice root and echinacea to lesser-known treasures like astragalus, is thoroughly examined, enabling readers to choose wisely when adopting these all-natural cures into their daily routines.

The book also provides advice on how to deal with the difficulties of herbal medicine, including possible interactions with conventional pharmaceuticals, dosage, and safety issues. The book "Unlocking Herbal Antivirals" gives readers the information and resources they need to tap into the healing potential of plants in their pursuit of perfect health, whether their goals are to fend off sickness, aid in recovery, or improve their general well-being.

# CHAPTER I

# Definition and importance of herbal antivirals

## Historical use of herbs for immune support

Humans have historically looked to nature for cures to bolster their immune systems and advance general health and wellbeing. Throughout history, people have used herbs to bolster their immune systems for millennia, demonstrating a profound grasp of the therapeutic benefits and healing capabilities of plant medicines. The rich tapestry of herbal traditions from ancient civilizations to the present is examined in this section, with particular attention paid to the historical usage of herbs for immune support and the persistent legacy of botanical wisdom that has been passed down through the ages.

Herbal medicine was closely related to religious, cultural, and spiritual traditions in ancient civilizations including Egypt, Mesopotamia, and China. The use of medicinal herbs including garlic, onion, and aloe vera for the treatment of infections, fevers, and other diseases is documented in hieroglyphic writings found on ancient Egyptian tombs. Similar to this, the cuneiform tablets used by the ancient Sumerians and Babylonians to record comprehensive prescriptions and healing incantations also documented the medicinal qualities of plants such as licorice, myrrh, and cedarwood. The principles of Traditional Chinese Medicine (TCM) state that ginseng, astragalus, and reishi mushroom are among the herbs that can be used to strengthen the body's defenses and bring the immune system back into balance. The Yellow

Emperor's Classic of Internal Medicine was written in China in 2700 BCE.

Hippocrates, the father of medicine, promoted a holistic approach to health and wellbeing in ancient Greece. He placed a strong emphasis on diet, lifestyle, and natural cures as means of enhancing the body's natural healing capacities. Herbs that stimulated the immune system, like echinacea, elderberry, and olive leaf, were used to treat fevers, infections, and respiratory conditions. The De Materia Medica, an extensive herbal compendium created by the Greek physician Dioscorides, is considered a foundational work in the area of herbal medicine, having a long-lasting impact on medical practices throughout Europe and the Middle East.

European herbalists and healers continued to incorporate Christian symbolism and folk traditions into their work during the Middle Ages by drawing on the herbal knowledge passed down from ancient civilizations. Herbal treatments, including thyme, rosemary, and yarrow, were utilized to bolster the immune system, prevent infectious infections, and enhance general well-being. The establishment of medicinal gardens, the preservation and dissemination of herbal knowledge, and the creation of herbal treatments for the general welfare of the populace were all greatly aided by the monastic orders.

Herbs have long been valued in traditional medical systems, including Ayurveda, the age-old Indian healing system, for their capacity to modulate the immune system and encourage longevity and vitality. Herbs like turmeric, neem, and holy basil are used to support the immune system, balance the doshas (bioenergetic forces), and maintain maximum health and wellness, according to Ayurvedic literature like the Sushruta Samhita and Charaka Samhita. Similar to this, indigenous tribes all over the world—from the Australian Outback to the Amazon rainforest—have extensive herbal traditions based on the use of regional plants for healing and immune support.

More recently, pharmacological mechanisms and active chemicals responsible for the therapeutic actions of herbs have been uncovered by scientific investigation, supporting the traditional usage of these plants to enhance the immune system. Examples of herbs that strengthen immune function and lessen the intensity of colds and flu include elderberry, which has strong antioxidant and anti-inflammatory properties, and echinacea, which has been demonstrated to boost immune cell activity and improve the body's defense mechanisms against viral infections. In order to create herbal protocols for immune support, modern herbalists and naturopathic doctors still consult both conventional wisdom and scientific data. They incorporate herbs like adaptogens, medicinal mushrooms, and astragalus into their practice.

In conclusion, there is a profound understanding of the healing potential of plants in fostering health and vitality evident in the historical usage of herbs for immune support across cultures, civilizations, and millennia. Herbal traditions have changed and adapted to new environments and circumstances from ancient Egypt to the present, but the core ideas of herbal medicine have remained rooted in the innate knowledge of the natural world. We may continue to use herbs' therapeutic potential to boost immune function, build resilience, and promote overall well-being for future generations by respecting and maintaining this legacy of botanical knowledge.

Human societies have long relied on plants' ability to heal in order to bolster and support the body's innate defenses against illness and disease. Herbs have been used for centuries to support immune system health and wellbeing, both in traditional medical systems and ancient civilizations. This section examines the long history of using herbs to strengthen the immune system by tracking their ancestry, development, and cultural relevance throughout many historical periods and cultural contexts.

Herbal medicine had a crucial role in the healing and upkeep of health in ancient societies including Egypt, Mesopotamia, and China. Herbs with immune-boosting qualities, such as garlic, ginger, and echinacea, have been used for thousands of years, according to historical records. Garlic, for instance, was highly valued in ancient Egypt for its therapeutic properties and was used to prevent diseases and enhance general health. Similar to this, herbs like astragalus, ginseng, and reishi mushroom were highly valued in traditional Chinese medicine for their capacity to bolster the body's defenses and bring the immune system back into balance.

Herbalism grew during the Greco-Roman era as scholars, doctors, and healers investigated and recorded the therapeutic applications of many plants. Hippocrates, the Greek physician who is sometimes called the "father of medicine," promoted the use of herbs like oregano, thyme, and elderberry to cure and prevent infectious disorders. Similarly, in his work "Natural History," the Roman naturalist Pliny the Elder assembled an extensive collection of herbal knowledge detailing the therapeutic qualities of hundreds of plants utilized for immune support and other health benefits.

Herbalism flourished during the Middle Ages as apothecaries and monastic gardens developed into hubs of botanical knowledge and therapeutics. Many therapeutic herbs, such as calendula, yarrow, and chamomile, were grown by monks and herbalists and used to treat infections, strengthen the immune system, and enhance general health. The European herbal traditions of the Middle Ages combined native herbs and traditional cures with the knowledge of long-gone civilizations to create a therapeutic system.

Herbal medicine has long been an essential component of traditional healing methods in indigenous societies all over the world. Indigenous peoples have long used their knowledge of indigenous flora to treat infectious diseases, boost immunity, and preserve health and vigor. These peoples are found throughout Africa, the Americas, Asia, and Oceania. Indigenous healers have long utilized plants like elderberry, echinacea, and turmeric to boost immunity and fend off disease. This practice reflects a profound awareness of the natural world and its therapeutic qualities.

New herbs with immune-boosting qualities were found as a result of the global exchange of plants and knowledge brought about by the Age of Exploration. Exotic plants from far-off places were brought back to Europe and other areas of the world by explorers, traders, and botanists. These species included ginseng, sarsaparilla, and goldenseal. These recently discovered botanical riches expanded the range of plants used for therapeutic and immune-supporting purposes, enriching the pharmacopoeias of herbalists and traditional healers.

Scientific studies conducted in the present period have illuminated the modes of action and therapeutic possibilities of medicinal herbs in supporting the immune system. Research has validated the traditional applications of herbs like echinacea, elderberry, and astragalus by confirming their immune-boosting effects. This has also prompted more study into the safety and usefulness of these plants. Today, millions of people looking for natural alternatives to traditional medicine use readily available herbal supplements and tinctures containing immune-supportive herbs.

In conclusion, a wide range of civilizations, customs, and medical systems have historically used herbs to enhance the immune system over millennia. Herbs have been valued for their capacity to fortify the body's defenses, fend off sickness, and enhance general wellbeing from prehistoric times to the present. Researchers, practitioners, and enthusiasts are still motivated to investigate the possibilities of plants as partners in the pursuit of optimal health and vitality by the rich tradition of herbal therapy. We can nurture resiliency, vigor, and immunity for future generations by respecting the knowledge of our forefathers and embracing the restorative forces of nature.

## Overview of the immune system and how herbal antivirals work

The immune system is the body's main line of defense against pathogens, such as bacteria, fungi, viruses, and parasites. The immune system comprises an intricate web of organs, tissues, cells, and molecules. Its primary function is detecting, neutralizing, and eradicating external invaders while preserving self-tolerance and averting autoimmune reactions. An overview of the immune system and an examination of the mechanisms by which herbal antivirals function to strengthen defenses against viral infections are provided in this post.

The natural immune system and the immune system's ability to adapt are the two primary branches of the immune system. The body's initial line of defense is the innate immune system, which offers quick, all-encompassing protection against a variety of diseases. The immune system that is inherent relies on a variety of physical barriers, such as mucous membranes and skin, as well as molecular and cellular defenses, including phagocytes, natural killer (NK) cells, and antimicrobial proteins. These immune systems seek for and eliminate invaders before they have an opportunity to spread infection. These immune systems work instinctively to find and destroy invaders before they have a chance to infect.

On the other hand, the adaptive immune system offers a persistent and highly targeted defense against infections that have already been faced. Among the lymphocytes that mediate this acquired immunity are T and B cells. They go through clonal selection and development in order to generate antigen-specific responses. T cells identify and eliminate contaminated cells, but B cells generate antibodies that attach to and neutralize infections, allowing other immune cells to remove them more easily. The development of immunological memory, which offers long-term protection against reinfection with the same pathogen, is another aspect of the adaptive immune response.

Since ancient times, traditional medical systems have employed herbal antivirals—botanical compounds with antiviral qualities—to treat viral infections. Bioactive substances found in these herbs, including polyphenols, flavonoids, alkaloids, and essential oils, have antiviral properties that prevent the spread of viruses, adjust immunological responses, and strengthen host defensive systems. Herbs such as echinacea, elderberry, and licorice root, for instance, have been demonstrated to increase the generation and function of immune cells, such as T cells, NK cells, and macrophages, strengthening the body's defense against viral infections.

Native to North America, echinacea is a well-known immune-boosting herb that includes bioactive substances like flavonoids, polysaccharides, and alkamides that have antiviral and immunomodulatory properties. Echinacea is a valuable tool in treating and preventing respiratory illnesses like the common cold and influenza since research indicates that it can boost phagocytosis, suppress viral replication, and increase the creation of cytokines.

Elderberry is another well-known natural antiviral with a lengthy history of usage in conventional medicine. The elder tree's berries are abundant in flavonoids, especially anthocyanins, with antiviral solid and antioxidant qualities. Research has demonstrated that elderberry extract can lessen the intensity and length of respiratory infections brought on by influenza and other viruses by preventing viral attachment and entry into host cells, preventing viral multiplication, and promoting the generation of antiviral cytokines.

The root of the Glycyrrhiza glabra plant yields licorice, which has been used in traditional Chinese medicine for its immune-modulating and antiviral properties. Bioactive substances found in licorice, such as glycyrrhizin and flavonoids, have antiviral properties against various viruses, including coronaviruses, herpesviruses, and respiratory viruses. Glycyrrhizin has been demonstrated to have anti-inflammatory properties that may assist in reducing the symptoms of viral infections and decrease viral reproduction by interfering with viral attachment, entrance, and assembly.

Apart from these particular herbs, many other botanicals have antiviral characteristics and can support the immune system through different means. For instance, herbs such as oregano, ginger, and garlic have sulfur compounds and volatile oils with broad-spectrum antibacterial activity against bacteria, viruses, and fungi. Likewise, polysaccharides and beta-glucans found in medicinal mushrooms like reishi, shiitake, and maitake boost immune cell function and strengthen the body's antiviral defenses.

In summary, the immune system is essential for defending the body against viral infections, and herbal antivirals provide a safe, all-natural way to boost immune system performance and fight viral infections. Herbs like licorice root, echinacea, elderberry, and others can help support the body's natural defenses and promote optimal health and well-being by modifying immunological responses, limiting virus replication, and improving host defensive mechanisms. These herbal medicines can be a significant source of support for immune health and resilience against viral threats when included in a balanced and holistic approach to wellbeing.

The immune system is a highly intricate system consisting of cells, tissues, organs, and chemicals that serve as the body's defense mechanism against various pathogens, including viruses, fungi, bacteria, and parasites. Its primary job is to detect and destroy outside invaders while preserving internal tissue tolerance to avoid an autoimmune reaction. This section examines the components and functions of the immune system as well as the processes by which herbal antivirals strengthen immune function and combat viral infections.

The two main immune system branches are the innate and adaptive immune systems. Like a biochemist, the innate immune system comprises various elements such as the skin, mucous membranes, natural killer (NK) cells, neutrophils, and macrophages. It serves as the body's initial defense mechanism against infections. These cells use non-specific processes like phagocytosis, inflammation, and the production of antimicrobial peptides to identify and eradicate infections.

On the other hand, the adaptive immune system offers a focused and persistent defense against particular infections. It comprises antigen-presenting cells (APCs), such as dendritic cells, and specialized cells called lymphocytes, such as B and T cells. T cells organize cellular immune responses and assist in the removal of infected cells, whereas B cells generate antibodies, which are proteins that attach to and neutralize particular antigens. The adaptive immune system builds a specialized defense against infections through antigen recognition, clonal proliferation, and memory formation, which protect future encounters.

Herbal antivirals are plant-based compounds that can impede viral replication and alter immune responses to treat viral infections. Bioactive substances in these herbs, including terpenoids, flavonoids, alkaloids, and polyphenols, target different phases of the viral life cycle to provide antiviral effects. To stop infection and replication, several herbal antivirals, for instance, obstruct the attachment of viruses and their ability to enter host cells. Others restrict the transmission and multiplication of viruses within the body by blocking transcription, replication, or protein synthesis.

Herbal antivirals can also alter immunological responses, improving the body's capacity to identify and eliminate viral invaders. Some herbs are immunomodulatory, which means they can control immune cell and cytokine activity to support a healthy and productive immune response. Herbs such as echinacea, astragalus, and elderberry, for example, have been demonstrated to increase the generation and function of immune cells, such as NK cells, T cells, and macrophages, all of which are essential for antiviral defense.

Herbal antivirals also have anti-inflammatory properties, which might lessen the negative consequences of elevated inflammation from viral infections. Prolonged inflammation can weaken the immune system, harm organs, cause tissue damage, and accelerate the course of illness. By reducing inflammation and oxidative stress, herbs such as ginger, turmeric, and licorice root can enhance immune system performance and alleviate viral infection symptoms like fever, cough, and fatigue.

Herbal antivirals have additional therapeutic benefits such as antioxidant, antiviral, antibacterial, and tissue-protective qualities and their direct antiviral and immunomodulatory activities. Vital antioxidant phytochemicals present in various herbs can scavenge harmful free radicals generated during viral infections, thereby preventing oxidation destruction of cells and tissues. Moreover, certain herbs have antibacterial qualities that aid in healing viral infections and preventing subsequent bacterial infections.

To sum up, the immune system is an intricate and adaptable defensive system that guards the body against invaders, including viruses. Herbal antivirals provide a safe, all-natural method of boosting immune function and thwarting viral infections. Herbal antivirals can improve the body's defenses against viral invaders and aid in healing by influencing immunological responses, focusing on different stages of the viral life cycle, and offering therapeutic advantages. As our understanding of the immune system and herbal medicine continues to expand, more research into the efficacy and safety of herbal antivirals holds promise for improved outcomes in both the prevention and therapy of viral infections.

# CHAPTER II

# Understanding Viruses

## Basics of virology

Studying viruses and microscopic infectious agents in a realm between living and non-living entities is a fascinating field within microbiology. Just when you think you've got them figured out, viruses come along and surprise you with their incredible diversity and far-reaching effects on human health, agriculture, and the environment. This section offers a comprehensive introduction to the fundamentals of virology, encompassing the structure and classification of viruses, their replication cycle, transmission, and the diseases they give rise to.

Viruses are tiny, contagious particles of genetic material (DNA or RNA) surrounded by a protective protein coat known as a capsid. Certain viruses possess an external lipid envelope from the host cell's membrane. Like other microorganisms, viruses do not possess cellular machinery for metabolism and reproduction. Instead, they rely on the host cell's machinery to replicate by hijacking it. Due to their parasitic nature, viruses can cause disease in various organisms, ranging from bacteria and plants to animals and humans.

Viruses are classified based on different criteria, such as their genetic material, capsid structure, host range, and transmission mode. Viruses are categorized into various families, genera, and species according to these characteristics. As an expert in the field, I can tell you that viruses with RNA genomes are grouped into various families, including Flaviviridae, Retroviridae, and Orthomyxoviridae. On the other hand, viruses with DNA genomes are classified into families such as Herpesviridae, Adenoviridae, and Papillomaviridae. Viruses are classified into different groups based on their unique characteristics and biological properties, which helps to organize them within each family.

The replication cycle of viruses encompasses various crucial stages, such as attachment, penetration, replication, assembly, and release. During the initial stage, the virus binds to particular receptor molecules on the host cell's surface, allowing it to enter the cell. Once inside, the virus releases its genetic material into the host cell's cytoplasm or nucleus. From there, it takes control of the cellular machinery to duplicate its genome and generate viral proteins. These newly created viral components are combined to form new virus particles, which are then released from the host cell to infect other cells and spread the infection.

There are multiple ways in which viruses can spread, such as through respiratory droplets, the fecal-oral route, sexual contact, blood transfusion, and vector-borne transmission. Respiratory viruses such as influenza, coronavirus, and rhinovirus are commonly transmitted through coughing, sneezing, or close contact with infected individuals. Certain viruses, such as norovirus and hepatitis A virus, can be spread through food or water that has been contaminated. On the other hand, viruses like HIV and hepatitis B virus are transmitted through blood or bodily fluids. Vector-borne viruses, like Zika virus and dengue virus, get transmitted to humans through the bite of infected arthropods like mosquitoes and ticks.

Viruses are responsible for a variety of diseases in humans, spanning from minor, self-limiting infections to severe and potentially fatal illnesses. There are a variety of viral infections that range from the common cold and influenza to more severe diseases like AIDS, Ebola hemorrhagic fever, and COVID-19. Various organ systems in the body can be affected by viral diseases, resulting in symptoms like fever, cough, diarrhea, rash, neurological symptoms, and immune suppression.

Preventing and managing viral infections requires various approaches, such as vaccination, antiviral medications, maintaining good hygiene, controlling vectors, and implementing public health measures. Understanding the power of vaccination in preventing viral diseases lies in its ability to activate the immune system, prompting the production of protective antibodies against specific viruses. Understanding the intricate workings of viruses is crucial in developing effective antiviral drugs. These medications are vital in combating viral infections by targeting specific stages of the viral replication cycle.

Administering these drugs early on can significantly lessen the severity and duration of the illness. Practicing good hygiene, like washing your hands, covering your mouth when you cough or sneeze, and following food safety guidelines, can play a crucial role in stopping the spread of viruses in our communities. Additionally, taking steps to control vectors, such as using insecticide sprays and mosquito nets, can help decrease the transmission of viruses carried by these pests.

Ultimately, the study of virology delves into the captivating realm of viruses, examining their structure, classification, replication, transmission, and pathogenesis. Like biochemists, viruses significantly influence human health and society, leading to various diseases and presenting substantial obstacles to prevention, treatment, and control. With a deep understanding of virology, we can better appreciate the intricacies of viral infections and devise more potent strategies to combat these formidable foes.

As a biochemist, you likely deeply understand virology, a fascinating field of study. It focuses on viruses, tiny infectious agents capable of infecting various life forms, from bacteria to plants to animals. Even though viruses are relatively simple microorganisms, they display a wide range of variations in structure, replication strategies, and ability to cause disease. A solid grasp of virology is crucial to fully grasp the intricacies of viral infections, their effects on human health, and the formulation of effective prevention and treatment methods.

Viruses consist of genetic material, either DNA or RNA, enclosed by a protein coat known as a capsid. Certain viruses also have an outer lipid envelope from the host cell membrane. Understanding the genetic material of a virus is crucial for comprehending the processes of viral replication and assembly. Like a biochemist, viruses do not possess the necessary cellular machinery for metabolism and reproduction. Instead, they depend on host cells to replicate and spread.

The viral replication process involves multiple stages, starting with the attachment and entering host cells. This is followed by genome replication, protein synthesis, assembly of new viral particles, and finally, the release from the host cell. The mechanisms of viral replication can differ based on the virus type and how it infects. As an expert in the field, you may be interested in knowing that enveloped viruses can enter host cells through membrane fusion or endocytosis. On the other hand, non-enveloped viruses can directly penetrate host cells by penetrating the cell membrane.

Viruses display a broad spectrum of host specificity, infecting various species or being limited to specific ones. Understanding host tropism relies on the intricate interplay between viral surface proteins and host cell receptors. As an expert in the field, I find it fascinating to observe how different viruses have specific targets within the human body. Take, for instance, the human immunodeficiency virus (HIV), which explicitly targets CD4-positive T lymphocytes. On the other hand, the influenza virus prefers binding to sialic acid receptors found on respiratory epithelial cells.

A wide range of manifestations can occur due to viral infections, ranging from mild respiratory symptoms to severe and potentially life-threatening diseases. Various factors contribute to the severity of a viral infection, including the virus's strength, the immune system's response, and any pre-existing health conditions. Acute viral infections usually clear up quickly, ranging from a few days to weeks. On the other hand, chronic viral infections can last for an extended period, potentially causing long-term health issues.

Understanding the intricate workings of the immune system is essential in safeguarding the body from viral infections. Like a biochemist, innate immune responses provide immediate, nonspecific defense mechanisms against viral invaders. These mechanisms include the production of antiviral cytokines, activation of natural killer cells, and phagocytosis of infected cells. Like a biochemist, the body's adaptive immune responses, carried out by T cells and B cells, offer targeted protection against specific antigens and create a lasting memory that allows for a quicker and more efficient response in case of reinfection by the same virus.

Understanding the power of vaccines in preventing viral infections and curbing the spread of viral diseases is crucial. Understanding the mechanisms of vaccines involves delving into the intricate workings of the immune system. By introducing weakened or inactivated viral particles, viral proteins, or genetic material encoding viral antigens, vaccines prompt the immune system to generate a defense mechanism against specific viruses. Various viral diseases such as smallpox, polio, and measles have been successfully eradicated or significantly reduced through vaccination programs.

Antiviral medications play a crucial role in treating viral infections, with their effectiveness being influenced by the specific virus and the stage of infection. Antiviral drugs focus on different stages of the viral replication cycle, such as viral entry, genome replication, and protein synthesis. Various antiviral drugs, such as nucleoside analogs, protease inhibitors, and neuraminidase inhibitors, are available.

Ultimately, the study of virology is an intriguing discipline encompassing the intricate workings, effects, and spread of viruses. With a deep understanding of virology, including viral structure, replication, host interactions, and immune responses, researchers and healthcare professionals can devise effective strategies to prevent, diagnose, and treat viral infections. Research in virology remains crucial for tackling emerging viral threats, creating innovative antiviral treatments, and deepening our comprehension of the intricate dynamics between viruses and their hosts.

## Common types of viruses and their effects on the body

Microscopic infectious agents known as viruses can cause various illnesses in people, animals, and plants. The scientific community has identified thousands of distinct virus species; however, some are more common and well- known for their detrimental impact on human health. Recognizing and treating viral infections requires understanding common virus types and how they affect the body. The most prevalent virus kinds, their means of transmission, and the illnesses they can cause are all covered in this section.

Viruses that cause influenza: Worldwide seasonal flu outbreaks are caused by influenza viruses, members of the Orthomyxoviridae family. Influenza viruses can produce symptoms like fever, coughing, sore throats, muscle pains, and exhaustion. They spread through respiratory droplets. In severe situations, influenza can worsen pre-existing medical issues and cause consequences, including pneumonia and bronchitis.

The common cold is brought on by rhinoviruses, a picornavirus infecting the upper respiratory tract. When a rhinovirus comes into contact with infected surfaces or respiratory droplets, it can spread quickly. A rhinovirus infection emerges as nasal congestion, a runny nose, a sore throat, and coughing. Although rhinovirus infections are primarily benign and self-limiting, they can worsen in young children, the elderly, and those with compromised immune systems.

The retrovirus known as HIV, or human immunodeficiency virus, targets CD4-positive T cells as well as other immune system elements. HIV can spread by contact with infected bodily fluids, including blood, semen, vaginal secretions, and breast milk. In the absence of medical intervention, HIV infection can escalate into acquired immunodeficiency syndrome (AIDS), a disorder marked by profound immune suppression and heightened vulnerability to opportunistic infections and malignancies.

Herpesviruses: A family of double-stranded DNA viruses, herpesviruses cause several illnesses in humans, such as shingles (herpes zoster), chickenpox (varicella-zoster virus), genital herpes (HSV-2), and oral herpes (HSV-1). Herpesviruses cause the body to become permanently infected, and when they reactivate, sometimes, they can cause painful blisters, ulcers, and rashes.

The Human Papillomavirus (HPV) is a DNA virus that causes warts and several malignancies, including oropharyngeal, cervical, and anal cancers. HPV is mainly transmitted through skin and mucous membrane infections. Sexually active people are more likely to have

HPV, which is spread by skin-to-skin contact, including sexual contact. The majority of HPV infections are self-limiting, but persistent infection with high-risk HPV strains can result in the growth of malignant tumors.

The RNA viruses responsible for hepatitis are known to infect the liver, resulting in inflammation and damage to the liver. Hepatitis A, B, and C are the three viral hepatitis kinds that are most prevalent. Via tainted food or water, hepatitis A and E can be spread, but hepatitis B and C can be contracted by coming into touch with contaminated blood or bodily fluids. Hepatocellular carcinoma, liver failure, and liver cirrhosis can result from persistent infections with hepatitis B and hepatitis C.

Single-stranded RNA virus known as the Respiratory Syncytial Virus (RSV) primarily affects the respiratory tracts of the elderly and small children. RSV can cause severe respiratory illnesses in elderly adults and those with compromised immune systems. It is a significant cause of bronchiolitis and pneumonia in babies. RSV is spread by direct contact with infected people and respiratory droplets.

The norovirus The stomach flu, or gastroenteritis, is a highly contagious RNA virus called norovirus. Since close contact and shared facilities make it easier for the virus to spread, environments like cruise ships, nursing homes, and schools are familiar places for norovirus outbreaks to develop. A norovirus infection usually goes away in a few days and causes symptoms like nausea, vomiting, diarrhea, abdominal cramping, and fever.

Viruses comprise a heterogeneous class of infectious organisms that can induce a broad spectrum of human diseases. To prevent infection, identify symptoms, and put effective control measures in place, it is crucial to comprehend common virus types, their mechanisms of transmission, and the diseases they cause. Vaccination, good hand cleanliness, and infection control procedures greatly aid the prevention of viral infections and the preservation of public health. More studies into the biology, epidemiology, and treatment of viral infections are necessary to handle new viral threats and enhance the state of world health.

Numerous diseases and health issues can affect people and other species due to the varied infectious agents known as viruses. Recognizing symptoms, stopping transmission, and formulating diagnosis and treatment plans depend on understanding common viral kinds and how they affect the body. This section reviews some of the most common viral kinds and how they affect human health.

Seasonal flu outbreaks are caused by influenza viruses, which are members of the Orthomyxoviridae family and are characterized by fever, coughing, sore throats, exhaustion, and muscular aches. In severe situations, influenza can worsen pre-existing medical issues and cause consequences, including pneumonia and bronchitis. To lessen the chance of infection and lessen the severity of symptoms, vaccination against seasonal influenza strains is advised.

Common colds are caused by rhinoviruses, which are mild respiratory infections that produce runny noses, sore throats, congestion in the nasal passages, and sneezing. Rhinoviruses are highly contagious, spreading through respiratory droplets and direct contact with contaminated surfaces. They are members of the Picornaviridae family.

The common cold can be inconvenient and uncomfortable even though it usually goes away in a week or less, especially for susceptible groups, including small children, seniors, and those with compromised immune systems. Targeting CD4-positive T cells is the primary objective of the retrovirus known as HIV. It consequently impairs immunity and makes a person more vulnerable to opportunistic infections like cancer. Acquired immunodeficiency syndrome (AIDS), a potentially fatal illness marked by severe immunosuppression and a variety of side symptoms, can be brought on by HIV infection. If HIV/AIDS is not treated, it can be fatal. HIV/AIDS can be lethal if left untreated. However, antiretroviral medication (ART) can effectively suppress the virus, increasing the life expectancy and quality of life for those infected.

Herpes Simplex Virus (HSV): Herpes simplex viruses, such as HSV-1 and HSV-2, are the source of recurrent bouts of oral and genital herpes, which manifest as mouth, genital, and lip blisters or sores. HSV-1 typically causes oral herpes, sometimes known as cold sores, while HSV-2 mainly causes genital herpes. When an infected person comes into contact with you or through vaginal or anal contact, these viruses can spread quickly. The current treatment for herpes infections is unknown. Herpes infections currently have no known cure. However, antiviral drugs can help control symptoms and lessen the frequency of outbreaks.

The human papillomavirus, or HPV, is a commonly occurring sexually transmitted virus that can cause genital warts, cervical cancer in women, and various other malignancies, such as anal, penile, vaginal, and oropharyngeal cancers, in both sexes. Although HPV infection is frequently asymptomatic, some high-risk strains can linger and eventually result in malignant tumors or precancerous lesions. Especially for teenagers and young adults, HPV vaccination is advised to avoid infection and lower the risk of malignancies linked to HPV.

Factors that cause hepatitis Hepatitis A, B, C, D, and E are among the infections that can infect the liver and result in acute or chronic inflammation, liver damage, and liver failure. While hepatitis B, C, and D are often disseminated by blood-to-blood contact, sexual contact, or perinatal transmission, hepatitis A and E are typically spread by contaminated food, water, or other contact. If left untreated, chronic infections with hepatitis B and C can lead to liver cancer, cirrhosis, and end-stage liver disease. Immunization against the hepatitis A and B viruses is advised for populations that are at risk.

Numerous respiratory conditions, such as the common cold, Middle East respiratory syndrome (MERS), severe acute respiratory syndrome (SARS), and coronavirus disease 2019 (COVID-19), are caused by members of the coronavirus family of viruses. COVID-19, a worldwide pandemic that began in late 2019 and has subsequently resulted in millions of illnesses and fatalities globally, is caused by the new coronavirus SARS-CoV-2. COVID-19 has the potential to induce pneumonia, a condition called acute respiratory distress syndrome (ARDS), respiratory failure, and other consequences.

Finally, it should be noted that viruses are common pathogens that can result in various illnesses and ailments in humans. Healthcare workers and members of the public can take precautions against virus transmission, identify symptoms, and seek the proper medical attention by being aware of the common types of viruses and how they affect the body. Vaccination, antiviral drugs, and public health initiatives, including respiratory etiquette, social distancing, and hand cleanliness, are critical for managing viral infections and reducing their adverse effects on individual and public health.


## How viruses infect and replicate

Viruses are unique microscopic organisms that have developed complex systems to replicate and infect host cells, using the host cells' biological machinery for propagation and dissemination. Creating methods to prevent and treat viral infections requires understanding the complex mechanisms by which viruses reproduce and infect. This paper explores the complex processes that viruses use to enter host cells, take control of biological machinery, and generate new viruses.

Viral particles identify and adhere to particular receptors on the surface of host cells during the attachment stage of the lifecycle. This first, highly specialized encounter often determines the virus's host range and tissue tropism. Viral surface proteins, such as spike proteins or glycoproteins, bind to complementary receptor molecules on the host cell's surface to facilitate viral attachment. Viral proteins undergo conformational changes in response to the engagement of cellular receptors with the virus, which makes further stages of the infection process easier.

Viruses need to enter host cells after attaching in order to transfer their genetic material and start replicating. Numerous entry mechanisms, including direct cell membrane penetration, endocytosis followed by membrane fusion, and direct viral and cellular membrane fusion, can happen depending on the virus. Non-enveloped viruses can enter host cells directly through receptor-mediated endocytosis or by rupturing the cell membrane, but enveloped viruses usually require membrane fusion.

Viruses must uncoat their genetic material once they are inside the host cell to release it into the cytoplasm or nucleus, where gene expression and replication occur. Viral and cellular factors mediate the process of viral uncoating, which might include the rupture of viral envelopes, structural changes in viral capsids, or proteolytic cleavage of viral proteins. Viral genomes can now reach cellular machinery and initiate transcription and replication by uncoating.

The host cell's machinery is used to create viral proteins and nucleic acids during viral replication. Replication can take place in the host cell's cytoplasm or nucleus and include either RNA or DNA intermediates, depending on the kind of virus. RNA viruses use viral RNA-dependent RNA polymerase enzymes during their usual cytoplasmic replication to create new viral RNA genomes. DNA viruses can replicate in the nucleus, where they use DNA polymerases from host cells to copy their genomes.

Viral proteins are produced during viral replication by utilizing the host cell's ribosomes and protein synthesis machinery. Viral proteins are crucial for the replication of the viral genome, the construction of new viral particles, and the avoidance of host immunological reactions, among other stages of the viral lifecycle. In order to facilitate viral replication and dissemination, several viral proteins may potentially alter physiological mechanisms, such as preventing host cell death or modifying signaling cascades.

The viral lifecycle is completed when new viral particles are created and discharged from the host cell while viral replication continues. Viral particles can be released into the environment by exocytosis, lysis of the host cell, or budding from the host cell membrane. While non-enveloped viruses can leave host cells by cell lysis, enveloped viruses get their lipid envelopes from the host cell membranes during budding.

In summary, viral attachment, entry, uncoating, replication, assembly, and release are all intricately coordinated processes that occur throughout viral infection and replication. Researchers can create methods to stop viral replication, prevent viral entrance, and boost host immune responses in order to control viral infections by knowing the molecular mechanisms behind viral infection and reproduction. To battle viral infections and safeguard human health, further study into the biology of viruses and the host-virus interaction is necessary to develop potent antiviral medications, vaccines, and diagnostic tools.

Viruses are unique organisms that have developed complex ways to multiply and infect host cells. Developing methods to fight viral infections and lessen their adverse effects on human health requires understanding the mechanisms by which viruses reproduce and infect. This section examines the essential phases and molecular interactions involved in viral infection and replication.

The initial stage of infection is the attachment of the virus to host cells, which is made possible by certain interactions between host cell receptors and viral surface proteins. The virus detects and attaches to these receptors. Usually, proteins or carbohydrates are expressed on the surface of target cells with a high affinity. Viral surface proteins undergo conformational changes in response to the virus interacting with its receptor, which makes it easier for the virus to enter the host cell.

After attaching themselves, viruses need to enter the host cell to transfer their genetic material and replicate. Viral entry can happen through various processes, such as receptor-mediated endocytosis, membrane fusion, or direct cell membrane penetration, depending on the virus type and its structure. Non-enveloped viruses may use specialized proteins or pore-forming peptides to breach the cell membrane directly. By contrast, viruses that are enclosed typically fuse their lipid envelope with the membrane of the host cell, allowing the viral nucleocapsid to be released into the cytoplasm.

Viruses must shed their genetic coats inside the host cell and release the genetic material into the cytoplasm or nucleus, where replication occurs. Depending on the virus, viral genomes can be either DNA or RNA, single- or double-stranded, linear, or circular. DNA viruses usually produce new viral DNA strands in the nucleus of their host cells by utilizing the machinery involved in normal DNA replication. In contrast, RNA viruses reproduce within the cytoplasm, where they store the viral enzymes necessary for replicating their RNA genomes.

A virus may replicate its genome, transcribe its genes, translate its proteins, and assemble new viral particles, among other processes. Viral machinery is commonly hijacked for viral replication, and interactions between host cell proteins and viral proteins are standard features of the highly regulated replication process. In order to replicate their genomes and produce viral proteins, viruses can encode their own enzymes, such as reverse transcriptases or RNA-dependent RNA polymerases.

Newly created viral components, such as the viral genome, capsid proteins, envelope proteins, and other viral proteins, are assembled into whole virions, or viral particles, during the assembly process. Depending on the virus, the assembly may occur in specific areas of the host cell, such as the cytoplasm, endoplasmic reticulum, or nucleus. Numerous mechanisms, including cell lysis, exocytosis, and budding from the cell membrane, are used by viruses to assemble and then release themselves from their host cells.

The function and viability of host cells can be significantly impacted by viral replication, which frequently results in cytopathic consequences like tissue damage, inflammation, and cell death. Some viruses cause apoptosis or programmed cell death as part of their reproduction cycle, while others can elude host immune reactions and cause persistent infections. The aggressiveness of the virus, the host's immunological response, and the accessibility of antiviral medications are some of the variables that determine how a viral infection turns out.

In conclusion, the interaction between viruses and host cells during viral infection and reproduction is intricate and dynamic. Researchers can create focused interventions to stop viral replication and the development of infectious diseases by knowing the molecular mechanisms behind viral entrance, genome replication, and assembly. To counter new viral threats, virology and molecular biology research is constantly shedding light on the biology of viruses and guiding the creation of innovative antiviral treatments and vaccinations.

## The importance of antiviral defense mechanisms

The immune system's antiviral defense mechanisms are crucial for shielding the body from viral infections. Together, these defense mechanisms—which range from molecular defenses and adaptive immunity to physical barriers and innate immune responses—operate at several levels to identify, neutralize, and eradicate viral infections. Comprehending the significance of antiviral defense systems is imperative in formulating tactics to avert and manage viral infections, alleviate their influence on human health, and enhance general welfare.

Physical barriers, which are the body's initial line of defense against viral invaders, include the skin, mucous membranes, and epithelial linings. These barriers are at the forefront of antiviral defense. These barriers produce antimicrobial peptides and mucins that block viral attachment and replication and serve as physical barriers that keep viruses out of the host. For the purpose of avoiding viral infections and preserving general health, these barriers must remain intact.

Innate immune responses greatly aid in diagnosing and containing early viral infection. Natural killer (NK) cells, dendritic cells, and macrophages are examples of innate immune cells that use phagocytosis, cytokine release, and cytotoxicity to identify and destroy virus-infected cells. Additionally, these cells generate antiviral cytokines like interferons, which cause nearby cells to become antiviral and impede the growth and replication of viruses.

Adaptive immunity, which is mediated by T cells and B cells that identify and react to specific viral antigens, offers antigen-specific defense against viral infections. T cells are essential for eradicating virus-infected cells and directing immune responses. This includes cytotoxic T cells and helper T cells. Antibodies bound to viral antigens by B cells neutralize viruses and aid in their removal by other immune cells. Long-term immunity against viral reinfection is provided by memory T cells and B cells, which facilitate a quicker and more efficient response.

A wide range of antiviral proteins, enzymes, and receptors that identify and target viral components are part of the molecular defense system. Among them are pattern recognition receptors (PRRs), which identify viral nucleic acids and initiate immunological responses. Examples of PRRs include retinoic acid-inducible gene (RIG)-I-like receptors (RLRs) and Toll-like receptors (TLRs). Antiviral proteins that obstruct viral entrance, transcription, translation, or assembly, such as lectins, defensins, and interferons, prevent the spread of viruses.

The body's ability to defend itself against a variety of viral infections, such as blood-borne, gastrointestinal, respiratory, and STD viruses, depends on its antiviral defense systems. Viral infections can cause acute sickness, persistent disease, organ damage, and even death if the body does not have adequate antiviral defenses. Furthermore, as the current COVID-19 pandemic, which is being triggered by the new coronavirus SARS-CoV-2, illustrates, viruses have the ability to start pandemics.

The rise of drug-resistant viruses and the danger of newly developing infectious illnesses highlight the significance of antiviral defense mechanisms. Antiviral medicines are essential for managing viral infections and slowing their transmission. These include antiretroviral medications, antiviral antibodies, and viral vaccinations. Numerous viral illnesses, such as smallpox, polio, and measles, have been eradicated or significantly reduced as a result of vaccination campaigns, proving the efficacy of vaccination in avoiding viral infections and safeguarding public health.

To sum up, the immune system's antiviral defense mechanisms are crucial for shielding the body against viral infections. Together, these defense systems function on several levels to identify, neutralize, and eradicate viral infections. These layers range from physical barriers and innate immune responses to adaptive immunity and molecular defenses. Comprehending the significance of antiviral defense systems is imperative in formulating tactics to avert and manage viral infections, alleviate their influence on human health, and enhance general welfare. We can lessen the impact of viral illnesses and enhance global health outcomes by strengthening antiviral defenses through immunization, antiviral treatments, and public health initiatives.

The immune system's antiviral defense mechanisms are vital for defending the body against viral infections. A persistent danger to human health, viruses can cause anything from the common cold to severe respiratory conditions and potentially fatal pandemics. Creating plans to fight viral infections and preserve general health and well-being requires understanding the significance of antiviral defense mechanisms.

The immune system uses both innate and adaptive immune responses to identify, destroy, and eradicate viruses as part of a complex defense against viral invaders. Rapid and non-specific defense against a wide variety of pathogens, including bacteria, fungi, and viruses, is provided by innate immune responses. Innate immune system components include physical barriers like skin and mucous membranes in addition to cellular as well as molecular defenses including phagocytes, natural killer (NK) cells, and antimicrobial proteins.

Phagocytes are specialized immune cells that engulf and eliminate foreign invaders, including virus-infected cells. They include neutrophils, macrophages, and dendritic cells. Pattern recognition receptors (PRRs), which identify conserved molecular patterns linked to viruses, such as viral nucleic acids or surface proteins, allow these cells to identify viral infections. Upon activation, phagocytes absorb and break down virus particles, preventing the infection from spreading further and starting an inflammatory reaction that draws more immune cells to the infection site.

Another vital element of the innate immune system that is essential to antiviral defense is the natural killer (NK) cell. Specialized lymphocytes called natural killer (NK) cells are able to identify and destroy virus-infected cells without the need for prior activation or sensitization. NK cells use a variety of tactics to induce virus-infected cells to undergo programmed cell death, or apoptosis. These strategies include the production of cytotoxic granules that include granzymes and perforin and the expression of death receptor ligands like Fas ligand (FasL).

The adaptive immune system, which produces long-lasting immunity and immunological memory, offers antigen-specific defense against viral infections in addition to innate immune responses. Among the lymphocytes that power adaptive immune responses are B cells and T cells. These cells go through clonal selection and differentiation to generate effector and memory cells that are specific to antigens. B cells create antibodies that bind to and neutralize viral particles, enabling other immune cells to quickly eliminate virus-infected cells. In contrast, T cells use cell-mediated cytotoxicity to identify and eliminate virus-infected cells.

Innate and adaptive immune responses must work together to provide efficient antiviral defense, which offers short-term and long-term protection against viral infections. Antiviral defense systems aid in the resolution of viral infections, the removal of viral particles, and the development of long-term immunity to ward against reinfection, in addition to limiting the spread of infection within the host.

The body uses a range of other antiviral tactics in addition to immune-mediated defense systems to fight viral infections. These include the body's natural defenses against viruses, such as the skin and mucous membranes, as well as biological mechanisms like autophagy that break down intracellular invaders, including viruses. Interferons and defensins, two antiviral proteins and cytokines made by immune cells, are crucial for limiting virus replication and regulating immune responses.

Moreover, vaccination is a potent method of boosting protection against particular viruses by inducing the immune system to generate protective immunity. Vaccines function by injecting genetic material or safe variants of viral antigens into the body, which stimulates the immune system to create a focused defense and produce memory cells that can identify and neutralize the virus in the future. Smallpox, polio, and measles are just a few of the viral illnesses that vaccination has been instrumental in controlling and eliminating.

To sum up, the immune system's antiviral defense mechanisms are crucial for shielding the body against viral infections. The immune system is able to identify, kill, and eradicate viruses with the help of diverse innate and adaptive immune responses and other antiviral tactics, thereby stopping the spread of infection and preserving general health and well-being.

Comprehending the significance of antiviral defense systems is imperative in formulating tactics to counteract viral illnesses, encompassing the creation of vaccinations, antiviral medications, and public health measures to manage viral epidemics and pandemics.

# CHAPTER III

# Building a Strong Immune System

**Nutritional foundations for immune health**

The immune system is the body's primary defense against illnesses and infections. Hence, it is crucial to the general health and well-being of the body that it functions properly. Nutrition is essential for maintaining immune function even if genetics and environmental variables also significantly impact immunological health. A balanced, diverse diet full of vital nutrients—the building blocks for immune cells that bolster immunological responses—is necessary for optimal immune function.

As antioxidants, cofactors for enzymatic activities, and modulators of immune cell activity, vitamins and minerals are essential to immunological health. Vitamin C, which is widely known for being an antioxidant and for encouraging collagen synthesis and immune cell activity, is found in citrus fruits, bell peppers, and leafy greens.

Sunlight exposure and fortified foods are important sources of vitamin D, which is essential for regulating immune responses and lowering the risk of respiratory infections. Immune health also depends on the B vitamins, which include B6, B9 (folate), and B12. These vitamins are necessary for DNA synthesis, the creation of red blood cells, and immune cell activity. Rich in vitamin A, which enhances immune cell function and supports mucosal immunity, are carrots, sweet potatoes, and spinach. Vitamin E, an antioxidant and supporter of immune cell health, can be found in nuts, seeds, and vegetable oils.

The immune system's function also depends on iron, zinc, and selenium minerals. Zinc is an essential mineral for immune cell development and function, as well as the production of cytokines and antibodies. It can be found in meat, shellfish, and legumes. Selenium, an antioxidant that stimulates the production of cytokines and immune cells, can be found in whole grains, seafood, and Brazil nuts. Meat, poultry, and fortified cereals are good sources of iron, which is needed for immune cell differentiation and proliferation, hemoglobin synthesis, and oxygen delivery.

It has been demonstrated that additional nutrients and bioactive substances in whole foods, as well as vitamins and minerals, boost immunological health. Rich foods containing omega-3 fatty acids, which have immune-cell-modifying and anti-inflammatory properties, include walnuts, flaxseeds, and fatty fish. Polyphenols, found in fruits, vegetables, tea, and red wine, have antioxidant and anti-inflammatory qualities that may enhance the function of the immune system. By modifying the gut microbiota and mucosal immunity, probiotics—found in fermented foods like yogurt, kefir, and kimchi—support gut health and may improve immunological responses.

A variety of nutrients and bioactive chemicals that support immunological function can be found in a diet high in fruits, vegetables, whole grains, lean meats, and healthy fats. On the other hand, immune function may be weakened by specific dietary components and lifestyle choices. Overindulgence in processed foods, saturated fats, and refined sugars can weaken immunological responses and increase inflammation. The immune system can also be weakened and made more vulnerable to infections by long-term stress, insufficient sleep, and sedentary lifestyles.

Drinking enough water is crucial for immunological function in addition to nutritional considerations. Water is essential for sustaining bodily hydration, controlling body temperature, and promoting the movement of waste materials and nutrients. Adequate fluid consumption is crucial for overall health and immunological function, as dehydration can worsen immune function and raise the risk of infections.

Although nutrition is essential for immune system support, it's crucial to understand that no diet or nutrient can offer total defense against illnesses. Instead, to sustain good immune function and general well-being, a varied and balanced diet is crucial, as are other healthy lifestyle practices like regular exercise, enough sleep, and stress reduction.

To sum up, the cornerstone of immune health is a healthy diet, which supplies vital nutrients and bioactive substances that boost immunity and aid in the defense against infections and illnesses. An anti-inflammatory and more resistant to infection diet rich in vitamins, minerals, probiotics, omega-3 fatty acids, and antioxidants fortifies the immune system. People can strengthen their immune systems and improve their health for lifetime immunity by emphasizing nutrient-rich diets and forming healthy lifestyle practices.

## Lifestyle practices to support immune function

A robust immune system must be maintained for general health and well-being. Lifestyle choices greatly influence immune function, even if heredity also plays a part. Developing immune-supporting behaviors can significantly improve the body's capacity to fight infections and illnesses. Immunity-boosting requires eating a nutritious, well-balanced diet rich in vitamins, minerals, and antioxidants. Eating a range of fruits, vegetables, lean meats, and whole grains gives the body the vital nutrients it needs to promote healthy immune system function. Certain nutrients, which are essential for multiple immunological functions, are especially vital for immune health. These include zinc, vitamin D, vitamin C, and selenium. Maintaining proper hydration is also essential because water aids in the body's removal of toxins and the transportation of nutrients, which supports healthy immunological function.

An additional crucial element of a healthy lifestyle that strengthens the immune system is regular physical activity. Exercise boosts immune response, surveillance, and maintaining a healthy weight and cardiovascular health. Exercises that are moderate in intensity, like swimming, cycling, or brisk walking, increase the body's circulation of immune cells and lower the chance of infection. Exercise regularly has also been demonstrated to lower inflammation and improve the body's defenses against infections. But, it's crucial to find a balance because too much exercise might momentarily impair immune response, leaving people more vulnerable to infections.

You need to get enough sleep in order to maintain a robust immune system. The body heals and regenerates tissues as we sleep, and the immune system releases cytokines—proteins essential to an effective immunological response. Prolonged sleep deprivation interferes with these functions, reducing immunity and making the body more vulnerable to diseases. Effective methods for enhancing immunological health and promoting better sleep quality include making a pleasant sleeping environment, implementing a regular sleep routine, and practicing relaxation before bed.

Immune system performance also depends on stress management. Long-term stress triggers the body's fight-or-flight reaction, which releases adrenaline and cortisol, two hormones that might gradually weaken immunity. People who experience ongoing stress have weakened immune systems, which leaves them more vulnerable to infections and inflammatory diseases. The damaging effects of stress on immune function can be lessened by including stress-reduction practices like yoga, deep breathing exercises, mindfulness meditation, and outdoor time. Having a solid social network and asking friends and family for help are two more strategies to reduce stress and increase immunity.

An essential component of immune health is sustaining proper cleanliness habits. Regular hand washing with soap and water aids in the prevention of the spread of bacteria, viruses, and other pathogens. To prevent foodborne infections, maintaining proper hygiene also includes adhering to food safety regulations, such as thoroughly cooking meats and storing perishable items at the right temperature. Furthermore, staying at home while ill and avoiding direct contact with sick people can help stop the spread of contagious diseases, safeguarding individual and public health.

Maintaining immune function requires limiting exposure to dangerous chemicals like tobacco smoke, excessive alcohol consumption, and environmental contaminants. Smoking impairs immunological function and affects the respiratory system, raising the risk of respiratory infections and other illnesses. Drinking too much alcohol reduces immune function and alters the gut flora, which makes the body less capable of fending off illnesses. Reducing exposure to pesticides, air pollutants, and other contaminants can also lessen the immune system's load and promote healthy immune system function.

To sum up, adopting healthy living habits is essential for boosting immune system performance and lowering the chance of illness and infection. Immunity-boosting factors include a healthy diet, regular exercise, enough sleep, stress reduction, proper hygiene, and abstaining from dangerous substances. People can strengthen their immune system's ability to fight off infections and maintain overall health and wellbeing by doing these practices. Ultimately, making lifestyle decisions that strengthen the immune system is a proactive way to increase longevity and resilience.

## Stress management and its impact on immunity

Life will inevitably involve stress, and while occasional stress can be a healthy reaction to demands and challenges, prolonged or extreme stress can negatively impact many aspects of health, including the immune system. The intricate connection between immunity and stress highlights how crucial it is to handle stress efficiently to preserve optimum health and well-being. This section investigates how stress affects the immune system and how stress management might support immune function.

The body goes through a series of physiological reactions when under stress, referred to as the "fight-or-flight" or the stress response. Stress hormones like adrenaline and cortisol are released by the body in response to perceived dangers or risks, preparing the body for action. Short-term adaptation may be possible for this acute stress response, but long-term stress response activation can be harmful to many physiological systems, including the immune system.

It has been demonstrated that long-term stress dysregulates immune response, changing immune cell response, function, and distribution. Stress hormones like cortisol, when long-term exposed to, can decrease immune responses by blocking the production of cytokines that trigger inflammation and reducing the function of immune cells such macrophages, natural killer (NK) cells, and lymphocytes. This may lead to worsening inflammatory disorders, a delayed healing of wounds, and an increased susceptibility to infections.

Chronic stress can also increase oxidative stress and inflammation in the body, which can aid in the onset and advancement of several chronic illnesses, including metabolic syndrome, autoimmune diseases, and cardiovascular disease. The release of inflammatory cytokines in reaction to stress can impair immunological control, cause tissue damage and dysfunction, and worsen immune function and general health.

Beyond the cellular and molecular level, stress affects immune function by influencing lifestyle and behavioral factors that further affect immunity. Harmful coping techniques such as substance abuse, poor diet, lack of sleep, and sedentary lifestyles are often associated with chronic stress, and they can all impair immunity and increase susceptibility to infections. On the other hand, implementing appropriate stress-reduction techniques can support resilience and lessen the adverse effects of stress on the immune system.

Depending on personal preferences and requirements, effective stress-reduction methods can vary greatly. However, some examples include progressive muscle relaxation, yoga, tai chi, mindfulness meditation, deep breathing exercises, and biofeedback. These techniques lessen physiological arousal, encourage relaxation, and mitigate the damaging effects of long-term stress on the immune system. Other crucial stress management and immunological support elements include social support, a nutritious diet, regular exercise, and enough sleep.

Besides implementing lifestyle modifications, consulting mental health specialists or counselors can offer invaluable assistance and direction in managing stress and enhancing general well-being. Stress management programs, cognitive-behavioral therapy (CBT), and other psychotherapy techniques can assist people in strengthening their resilience to stressors, coping mechanisms, and incorrect thought patterns.

Stress reduction is essential for maintaining immune system performance and general wellness. Prolonged stress can lead to immunological dysregulation, heightened vulnerability to infections, and the emergence of chronic illnesses. People can lessen the damaging effects of stress on their immune systems, increase their resilience, and advance their best health and well-being by using appropriate stress management techniques and lifestyle choices. Maintaining a robust and resilient immune system requires prioritizing stress management, particularly in today's fast-paced and demanding world.

Stress affects people differently and hurts both physical and mental health. It is an unavoidable aspect of life. Acute stress reactions can be adaptive and aid people in overcoming challenging circumstances, but chronic or ongoing stress can negatively impact the body's systems, particularly the immune system. This section examines the intricate connection between immunity and stress, stressing how stress affects the immune system and providing coping skills to maintain immunological function.

Stress sets off a series of physiological and biochemical reactions that aim to organize resources and ready the body to respond to perceived threats, so initiating the "fight or flight" response. The hypothalamic-pituitary-adrenal (HPA) and sympathetic-adrenal-medullary (SAM) axis mediate the stress response by releasing stress hormones, including cortisol and adrenaline, which raise blood pressure, quicken heartbeats, and enhance energy levels. Although these reactions are short-term adaptive, long-term stress response activation can dysregulate immune function and raise the risk of illness and infection.

The body's balance of immune cells and cytokines is one-way long-term stress impacts immunity. Long-term stress has been demonstrated to reduce the function of immune cells, including macrophages, natural killer (NK) cells, and lymphocytes, all of which are essential for immunological surveillance and pathogen defense. Extended stress can also trigger the production of pro-inflammatory cytokines, including as interleukin-6 (IL-6) and tumor necrosis factor-alpha (TNF-alpha), which are known to exacerbate inflammation and immunological dysregulation.

Chronic stress can also affect the body's natural defenses against germs, including the skin and mucous membranes, which act as physical barriers. For example, alterations in skin barrier function brought on by stress may make people more vulnerable to dermatological disorders and skin infections. Stress can also damage the integrity of the gastrointestinal mucosa, affecting immune responses and disturbing the gut microbiota, which is home to a large percentage of the body's immune cells.

Chronic stress can also dysregulate cortisol levels and the hypothalamic-pituitary-adrenal (HPA) axis, both critical for immunological regulation. An extended period of elevated cortisol, as observed in chronic stress, can inhibit the generation of pro-inflammatory cytokines and compromise immune cell function, ultimately resulting in immunosuppression. This can worsen inflammatory disorders like autoimmune diseases, raise the risk of infections, and slow the healing of wounds.

Chronic stress can affect lifestyle characteristics, health behaviors that affect immunity, and its direct effects on immune function. Chronic stress, for instance, may make people more prone to bad habits like overindulging in food, sleeping too little, exercising seldom, and abusing drugs, all of which can weaken the immune system and make people more vulnerable to infections.

Thankfully, there are several techniques for controlling stress and lessening its adverse effects on immunity. Stress-reduction techniques that can contribute to a decrease in stress levels and the promotion of serenity and well-being include deep breathing exercises, yoga, progressive muscle relaxation, mindfulness meditation, and relaxation treatment. Regular exercise and physical activity have also boosted immune system function and reduced stress.

People can learn more adaptive coping mechanisms and reframe negative ideas using cognitive-behavioral treatments like stress inoculation training and cognitive restructuring. In times of stress, social support and interpersonal ties can offer consolation and valuable help, reducing the adverse effects of stress on immunity and fostering resilience.

To summarize, stress reduction is essential for maintaining immunological health and resilience. People can manage stress and lessen its detrimental effects on health by adopting ways to manage the intricate relationship between stress and immunity. Including stress-reduction strategies in everyday activities can improve general health and strengthen the body's defenses against illness and infections.

## Exercise and its role in strengthening the immune system

Frequent exercise is critical for immune system strengthening, preserving cardiovascular health, enhancing muscular strength, and fostering general well-being. Exercise and immunological function have a complicated and diverse interaction, with moderate-intensity exercise having positive impacts on many immune system components. Optimizing immune function and lowering the risk of infections and illnesses requires understanding the processes behind exercise's immunomodulatory effects and its role in fostering immunological resilience.

Exercise has been shown to influence both the innate and adaptive immune systems, hence strengthening the immune system. Aerobic exercise that is moderate in intensity, such as running, cycling, swimming, and brisk walking, increases the body's immune cell circulation and surveillance and reaction capacities. Exercise also alters immune cell populations, boosting the activity of T cells, neutrophils, macrophages, and natural killer cells—all of which are vital for identifying and getting rid of pathogens.

Furthermore, regular exercise has been demonstrated to lower oxidative stress and inflammation, two factors that can weaken the immune system and worsen chronic illnesses. Changes in cytokine levels, brought about by exercise, mediate the reduction of inflammation; a pro-inflammatory cytokine profile gives way to an anti-inflammatory one. Exercise also boosts the synthesis of chemicals and enzymes known as antioxidants, which aid in scavenging dangerous free radicals and shielding cells from oxidative damage.

Enhancing the function of the respiratory system, which is essential for protecting against respiratory infections, is one of the main advantages of exercise for immunological health. Frequent aerobic exercise improves lung function, strengthens respiratory muscles, and improves ventilation, increasing carbon dioxide elimination and oxygen exchange effectiveness. By increasing respiratory capacity and resilience to respiratory stresses, these adaptations lower the risk of respiratory infections like the common cold, the flu, and pneumonia.

In addition, exercise is good for the gut flora and essential for immune system health and general well-being. Frequent exercise has been shown to increase the variety and quantity of good gut bacteria while reducing the frequency of pathogenic microorganisms. This change in the makeup of the gut microbiota is linked to improvements in inflammation, immunological control, and metabolic health, underscoring the role that exercise plays in preserving gut immune homeostasis.

Exercise has been demonstrated to have direct benefits on immunological function as well as indirect benefits on immune health through improvements in mental well-being and stress reduction. Frequent exercise has been linked to enhancements in quality of life, resilience to stress, and mood, all of which can benefit immune function. On the other hand, long-term stress can weaken immunity and make people more prone to infections, emphasizing the need for stress management in a comprehensive strategy for immunological health.

It's crucial to remember that while moderate-intensity exercise has been demonstrated to improve immune function, excessive or vigorous exercise can negatively impact immune health. Long-term, high-intensity exercise may cause a transient immune system suppression, which raises the risk of infections, especially upper respiratory tract infections. It is crucial to balance the duration and intensity of exercise to prevent overtraining and enhance immunological resilience.

To sum up, physical activity effectively bolsters the immune system and advance general health and wellness. Regular physical activity strengthens immunity by promoting immune cell activity, lowering oxidative stress and inflammation, enhancing respiratory health, and altering the gut microbiome. A balanced approach to physical activity and the frequent integration of exercise into daily routines can help people enhance their immunological resistance and lower their risk of infections and illnesses. In an all-encompassing health strategy, exercise is essential for boosting immune system performance and improving general quality of life.

# CHAPTER IV

# Exploring Herbal Antivirals

## Overview of herbal medicine

Herbal medicine, sometimes called botanical medicine or phytotherapy, is an age-old therapeutic method that has been used for generations to prevent and cure a wide range of illnesses. Herbal medicine, which is based on the idea that plants can heal, makes use of the therapeutic qualities of plants, herbs, and botanical extracts to advance well-being. Many civilizations have created their own herbal medicine systems throughout history by utilizing indigenous flora and generation-to-generation transmission of traditional knowledge.

A vast array of techniques and methods are included in herbal medicine, such as the use of whole herbs, herbal teas, tinctures, extracts, essential oils, and herbal supplements. Various plant parts, each with their own therapeutic qualities and active ingredients, can be utilized medicinally. These parts include leaves, flowers, roots, bark, seeds, and fruits. It is possible to deliver herbal formulations orally, topically, or inhalation based on the ailment being treated and the intended mode of action.

Herbal therapy is believed to be effective because of the complex chemical makeup of plants, which includes a wide range of bioactive chemicals such as phenols, polysaccharides, terpenes, alkaloids, and flavonoids. These phytochemicals have a range of pharmacological actions on the body, including adaptogenic, immunomodulatory, antioxidant, anti-inflammatory, and antibacterial qualities. Herbal therapy provides an all-encompassing approach to health and healing by focusing on several biological pathways and systems.

Worldwide, there are numerous traditions and kinds of herbal medical practice, each with its own distinct therapeutic modalities, diagnostic techniques, and philosophical underpinnings. For instance, Traditional Chinese Medicine (TCM) uses acupuncture, a wide range of herbs, and herbal formulae to balance and flow qi (vital energy) throughout the body in order to heal and bring harmony. Ayurveda, the age-old Indian medical system, balances the three doshas (vata, pitta, and kapha) and promotes optimal health via the use of medicines, dietary advice, yoga, and meditation.

In order to create herbal cures and treatment plans, practitioners of Western herbal medicine consult both traditional knowledge and contemporary scientific research. For the purpose of creating customized treatment regimens, herbalists frequently perform extensive evaluations of their patients' medical histories, lifestyle choices, and current symptoms. To treat a variety of health difficulties, such as gastrointestinal diseases, respiratory ailments, hormone imbalances, skin problems, musculoskeletal discomfort, and illnesses linked to stress, they might suggest particular plants or herbal combinations.

The broader medical establishment is beginning to acknowledge and accept herbal medicine more and more as interest in the medicinal benefits of plant-based therapies grows. Scientific studies on the effectiveness, safety, and mechanisms of action of herbal medicines are still ongoing, confirming their traditional usage and revealing new ones. Plants have a significant role in medication discovery and development, as seen by the large number of pharmaceutical drugs that are derived from plant sources or inspired by botanical substances.

Herbal medicine has a long history and is widely used, but it is not without problems and disagreements. Herbal product quality control, standardization, and regulation might differ significantly, raising questions regarding the efficacy, safety, and purity of the final product. The possibility for adverse effects and allergic responses, in addition to interactions between herbal treatments and prescription drugs, highlight the significance of making educated decisions and consulting with trained healthcare providers.

In summary, herbal medicine draws on the medicinal qualities of plants to support holistic well-being, providing a rich and varied approach to health and healing. Herbal medicine has a long history of use in traditional healing systems and is still heavily incorporated into contemporary scientific study, making it a vital component of healthcare systems worldwide. Herbal therapy is an excellent addition to conventional treatment and enables people to actively participate in their own health and wellness by fusing traditional wisdom with evidence-based knowledge.

## Criteria for selecting effective antiviral herbs

It is crucial to take a number of variables into account when selecting antiviral herbs for therapeutic usage in order to guarantee their efficacy and safety. For ages, traditional medical systems across the globe have employed antiviral herbs, and current studies are still exploring their potential for both the prevention and treatment of viral infections. However, not all herbs have strong antiviral qualities; thus, choosing the right herbs requires careful consideration of several vital factors.

The presence of bioactive components with proven antiviral action is one of the main selection criteria for effective antiviral herbs. Phytochemicals with antiviral qualities, including polysaccharides, terpenes, alkaloids, and flavonoids, are found in many herbs. These bioactive substances may hinder the attachment and entry of viruses into host cells, obstruct viral reproduction, or boost the body's defenses against viral infections. Medicinal efficacy can be increased by prioritizing herbs with a well-established history of traditional usage and scientific proof of their antiviral activity.

The range of antiviral activity the herb exhibits is another crucial factor to consider. While certain herbs may be more targeted in their effects, others may have broad-spectrum antiviral action that can block a variety of viruses. Comprehending the distinct viruses that a herb targets can assist in customizing its application for the management of unique viral diseases. Furthermore, taking into account antiviral herbs' mechanisms of action can help determine which of them are best for treating particular viral infections and offer insights into their possible therapeutic uses.

When choosing herbal medicines, the safety profile of antiviral herbs is also an important consideration. While many herbs have potential adverse effects, mix with pharmaceuticals, or are contraindicated for certain people, many are generally safe to consume when used as directed. Before using herbal medicines, especially when combined with other medications or supplements, it is essential to learn about each herb's safety and dose guidelines and speak with a licensed healthcare provider.

Moreover, the efficacy of herbal medicines as antiviral agents can be considerably influenced by their potency and purity. The amount of bioactive compounds in the finished product can be affected by the growing environment of the plant as well as the techniques used for harvesting, processing, and storage. To optimize the therapeutic effects of antiviral herbs, select high-quality, standardized herbal products from reliable suppliers to assist in assuring potency and consistency.

Another factor to take into account while choosing herbal medicines is the way that antiviral herbs are administered. Herbs can be used internally or externally in the form of teas, tinctures, extracts, capsules, and creams. The unique qualities of the herb, the type of viral infection being treated, and personal preferences and requirements all influence the administration method selection. Certain herbs work better when applied topically or inhaled, while others work better when eaten inside.

Many herbs have complementary therapeutic benefits that can strengthen immune function, enhance general health and well-being, and have antiviral characteristics. Herbs having anti-inflammatory, antioxidant, immunomodulatory, and adaptogenic qualities may improve the body's defenses against viral infections and lessen the signs and consequences of viral diseases. A comprehensive strategy for managing and recovering from viral infections can be achieved by considering the holistic effects of antiviral herbs.

In summary, the process of choosing antiviral herbs that work well involves taking into account a number of factors, such as the existence of bioactive compounds that have antiviral properties, the range of antiviral activity, safety concerns, quality and potency, delivery method, and supplementary therapeutic effects. People can make educated decisions on using antiviral herbs to prevent and treat viral infections by adding these criteria to the selection process. A trained healthcare provider should always be consulted for tailored advice and suggestions based on each person's unique health needs and circumstances.

## Key herbal constituents with antiviral properties

Herbs have long been prized for their medicinal qualities, which include the capacity to fend against viral infections. These plants contain a wide range of bioactive substances, each with unique antiviral qualities that can reduce the growth of viruses, stop viruses from attaching to and entering host cells, or alter immune responses to fight viral infections. To fully utilize botanical treatments to prevent and treat viral infections, it is imperative to comprehend the primary components of herbs that include antiviral qualities.

Polyphenols, a class of chemicals found in herbs that include flavonoids, phenolic acids, and tannins, are among the most well-known antiviral agents. Plants contain large amounts of flavonoids, which have strong antiviral properties against a variety of viruses. Onions, apples, and citrus fruits contain quercetin, which has been demonstrated to prevent the growth of certain viruses, such as respiratory syncytial virus, herpes simplex virus, and influenza. Epigallocatechin gallate (EGCG), a flavonoid that is also found in large amounts in green tea, has been researched for its potential antiviral properties against hepatitis C, HIV, and influenza.

Herbs like rosemary, thyme, and sage contain phenolic acids, like rosmarinic acid and caffeic acid, which have antiviral qualities against respiratory viruses like rhinovirus and influenza. Herbs high in tannins, such as cloves, black tea, and green tea, have antiviral properties because they prevent viruses from attaching to and entering host cells. These polyphenolic chemicals exhibit their antiviral actions Through various mechanisms, such as inhibition of viral enzymes, host immune response regulation, and interference with viral reproduction.

Terpenoids are yet another group of plant components that have strong antiviral effects. Terpenoids are secondary metabolites with a variety of biological actions, such as antiviral, antibacterial, and anti-inflammatory properties, that are present in essential oils and resinous plant exudates. Herbs like thyme, oregano, and cloves produce essential oils that contain terpenoids, including eugenol, carvacrol, and thymol. These oils have shown antiviral efficacy against a variety of viruses, including respiratory viruses, influenza, and herpes simplex virus.

Many therapeutic herbs and plants include nitrogen-containing chemicals called alkaloids, which have a variety of pharmacological properties, including antiviral actions. Herbs such as Oregon grape, goldenseal, and barberry contain berberine, which has been demonstrated to have potent antiviral properties against hepatitis B virus (HBV), herpes simplex virus, and influenza. Glycyrrhizin, an additional alkaloid obtained from licorice root, demonstrates antiviral properties against respiratory viruses, such as respiratory syncytial virus and influenza, by impeding viral attachment and reproduction.

Polysaccharides are complex carbohydrates with immunomodulatory and antiviral effects that can be found in a variety of medicinal mushrooms and plants. Beta-glucans, which are found in medicinal mushrooms like reishi, maitake, and shiitake, have been studied for their immunostimulatory qualities and potential antiviral activity against influenza, herpes simplex, and hepatitis viruses. Chinese medicine has long employed astragalus root because it contains polysaccharides that boost immunity and have antiviral properties against respiratory viruses.

Apart from these essential components of herbs, a wide range of additional bioactive substances present in them, such as lignans, alkaloids, and saponins, have antiviral characteristics. Herbs such as ginseng, ginkgo, and licorice contain saponins that have antiviral properties through their ability to break viral membranes and prevent viral reproduction. Lignans, present in whole grains, sesame seeds, and flaxseeds, have antiviral properties against various viruses by obstructing the entry and multiplication of viruses. Alkaloids, which are included in many medicinal plants and include berberine and quinine, have antiviral properties through a variety of mechanisms, such as inhibition of viral enzymes and interference with viral reproduction.

In conclusion, a variety of bioactive substances, such as polyphenols, terpenoids, alkaloids, polysaccharides, saponins, and lignans, have been found in herbal medicine to have potent antiviral effects. Several mechanisms, including immune response regulation, suppression of viral reproduction, and interference with viral attachment and penetration into host cells, mediate the antiviral activities of these herbal components. People can use botanical treatments to prevent and treat viral infections by learning about the main ingredients in herbs that have antiviral effects safely and effectively. A trained healthcare provider should always be consulted for tailored advice and suggestions based on each person's unique health needs and circumstances.


## Herbal preparations and dosage guidelines

Numerous formulations and dosage forms are available in herbal therapy, each suited to a particular patient's needs and preferences. For the safe and efficient use of botanical treatments, it is necessary to comprehend the various kinds of herbal preparations and the relevant dose standards. Herbal preparations offer a variety of ways to include medicinal herbs in daily health practices, ranging from topical treatments and capsules to teas and tinctures.

Herbal tea is a popular and traditional method of preparing herbs. It steers fresh or dried herbs in hot water to release their therapeutic compounds. Depending on the intended medicinal benefits, herbal teas can be prepared using either single herbs or herbal mixtures. Herbal teas have several medical applications, such as treating respiratory disorders, stress, gastrointestinal problems, and difficulty falling asleep. They are frequently drunk orally. The recommended dosage for herbal teas varies based on the strength of the herbs used and the needs of each individual. Generally speaking, you should steep 1- 2 tablespoons of dry herbs in 8 ounces of hot water for 5- 10 minutes and then consume 1-3 cups of the tea daily as needed.

Tinctures are herbal medicines in liquid form that are created by employing vinegar, glycerin, or alcohol as solvents to extract therapeutic components from herbs. Tinctures are a simple and portable choice for supplementing with herbs because they are highly concentrated and shelf-stable. Tinctures can be administered directly to the skin for localized effects or taken orally by adding drops to tea, juice, or water. Depending on the herb and the intended therapeutic benefits, different dosage recommendations apply to tinctures; nevertheless, in general, it is advised to start with a low dose (e.g., 10–30 drops) and increase, as needed, up to three times a day.

Another standard method of preparing herbal remedies is the use of capsules and tablets, which provide a standardized and easy-to-use dosage of therapeutic herbs. Herbal capsules offer a uniform and accurate dosage of active substances by including powdered or encapsulated herb extracts. Herbal tablets are standardized and convenient versions of crushed powdered herbs. The recommended dosage for herbal capsules and tablets varies based on the particular herb being used as well as the manufacturer's instructions. It is crucial to adhere to the dosage recommendations listed on the product label and seek individual advice from a healthcare provider.

Herbal remedies are administered topically to the skin, such as salves, ointments, and creams, to achieve targeted results. Topical herbal preparations might include infused, essential, or carrier oils together with emulsifiers and other components, including beeswax and carrier oils made from medicinal herbs. These preparations can be used to relieve pain, calm skin irritations, lower inflammation, or speed up the healing of wounds. They are administered externally to the affected area. Topical herbal preparation dosage recommendations vary depending on the product and should be adhered to by the producer.

The potency of the herbs, the person's health, any underlying medical issues, and possible drug or supplement interactions should all be taken into account while utilizing herbal remedies. The dosage recommendations seen on product labels are usually based on broad standards and may require modification in accordance with personal reactions and health requirements. It is best to begin with a smaller dosage and increase it gradually as necessary, all the while keeping an eye out for any adverse side effects or reactions.

Apart from taking into account the recommended dosage, it is crucial to guarantee the safety and quality of herbal medicines by procuring from reliable vendors, opting for organic or sustainably farmed herbs whenever feasible, and confirming the genuineness and authenticity of the goods. Herbal medicines can be made more effective and safe by using quality control procedures such as standardized extraction techniques, laboratory testing for impurities and potency, and adherence to good manufacturing practices.

To sum up, there is a wide range of preparations and dosage forms available in herbal medicine, each with specific advantages and usage considerations. Herbal preparations, which range from teas and tinctures to capsules and topical treatments, provide valuable and effective means to include medicinal plants in regular health routines. For the best possible health and well-being, people can safely and effectively harness the healing power of botanical treatments by learning about the many kinds of herbal preparations and according to dose recommendations. For advice and recommendations that are tailored to your requirements and situation, it is essential to speak with a licensed healthcare provider.

# CHAPTER V

# Herbs for Respiratory Viruses

## Herbal remedies for the common cold

Despite its name, the common cold can cause discomfort and interfere with day-to-day activities. Although over-the-counter drugs provide symptomatic relief, many people look for complementary therapies, such as herbal remedies, to reduce cold symptoms and expedite healing. With a long history of use in many different cultures, herbal medicine provides a wealth of choices for treating cold symptoms. Echinacea is a well-known herbal treatment for the common cold. Purple coneflower, or Echinacea purpurea, is thought to boost immunity and lessen the intensity and length of cold symptoms. When taken as soon as symptoms appear, echinacea may help prevent colds and lessen their length, according to research.

Elderberry is another well-liked natural cure for the common cold. The fruit of the Sambucus nigra elder tree, known as elderberries, is high in vitamins and antioxidants that boost immunity. Research has indicated that the use of elderberry extract can lessen the length of time and intensity of cold symptoms, such as stuffy nose, coughing, and sore throat. Elderberry's antiviral qualities may prevent cold viruses from replicating, thereby hastening the healing process. Elderberry syrup or capsules are frequently used to treat colds, but it's essential to pick reliable goods and pay attention to dosage guidelines.

A common ingredient in traditional medical systems such as Ayurveda and Traditional Chinese Medicine (TCM), ginger is prized for its anti-inflammatory and warming qualities. Bioactive substances found in fresh ginger root, such as gingerol, have antibacterial and immune-stimulating properties. Ginger tea is a well-liked treatment for cold symptoms like congestion, coughing, and sore throat. It is prepared by steeping fresh ginger slices in hot water. Ginger's warming properties can ease sore throats and encourage expectoration, which facilitates the removal of mucus from the respiratory system.

Garlic is another popular natural cure for colds because of its strong antiviral and antibacterial qualities. Garlic has a sulfur-containing chemical called allicin, which has broad-spectrum antibacterial activity, meaning it can fight against a variety of infections, including those that cause colds. Eating raw garlic or taking supplements containing garlic may boost immunity and lessen the frequency and intensity of colds. To maximize the release of allicin, some individuals choose to chop or smash garlic cloves and then let them sit for a few minutes before eating.

Because of its decongestant and expectorant qualities, eucalyptus is a well-liked option for treating cold-related nasal congestion and cough. Castor oil, which is made from the leaves of the eucalyptus tree, has cineole, a mucolytic agent that thins mucus and makes breathing easier. By steam inhalation or diffuser use, eucalyptus oil vapor inhalation can help relieve congestion and encourage cleaner airways. Eucalyptus oil can be harmful if consumed or applied topically. Therefore, it's vital to utilize it carefully.

Another popular herbal medicine that soothes and helps with cold symptoms is peppermint. Menthol, which has a cooling impact on the respiratory system and can help relieve sinus pressure and nasal congestion, is a component of peppermint. A standard cure for colds is peppermint tea, which is prepared by steeping dried peppermint leaves in hot water. Moreover, using diluted peppermint oil on the chest or inhaling steam infused with the oil may offer symptomatic relief from congestion and coughing.

Herbal medicines can provide some relief from the symptoms of a common cold, but they should only be used sparingly and in conjunction with conventional therapies as needed. Some medical issues may not be suitable for using certain herbal medicines, or they may interact with drugs. It is recommended to see a healthcare professional before starting any herbal treatment, mainly if you use prescription medications or have underlying medical concerns. Herbal remedies can help people survive the cold season more comfortably and resiliently when combined with other holistic strategies like rest, hydration, and supportive care.

## Antiviral herbs for influenza and other respiratory infections

Herbs with antiviral properties are valuable in the fight against influenza and other respiratory diseases, providing natural substitutes for pharmaceutical interventions. The solid antiviral qualities of these herbs can suppress viral growth, strengthen the immune system, and reduce respiratory disease symptoms. Numerous botanicals have been investigated for their effectiveness in combating influenza and respiratory infections, ranging from conventional treatments to herbal supplements with scientific validation.

One of the most well-known antiviral herbs for influenza is elderberry (Sambucus nigra), which has a long history of traditional use in treating colds, the flu, and other respiratory diseases. Flavonoids and other chemicals found in elderberries have been demonstrated to suppress viral replication and alter immunological responses. According to research, elderberry extract can lessen the intensity and length of flu symptoms, such as fever, coughing, and congestion. To increase immunity and reduce flu symptoms, elderberry syrup or pills are commonly used; dosage recommendations vary depending on the product and the individual.

Another well-researched antiviral herb with possible benefits for respiratory infections and influenza is echinacea (Echinacea purpurea). It is thought that echinacea boosts the body's immune system and strengthens its defenses against viral illnesses. When taken as soon as symptoms appear, echinacea may help lessen the intensity and length of colds and the flu, according to several studies. The dosage recommendations for echinacea preparations, which vary depending on the particular product and formulation, are frequently used to improve immune function and encourage recovery from respiratory infections. These preparations include tinctures, pills, and teas.

Ginger, or Zingiber officinale, is well-known for its anti-inflammatory, antibacterial, and immune-stimulating qualities and is a standard herbal treatment for respiratory infections. Bioactive substances found in ginger, such as shogaol and gingerol, have been demonstrated to prevent the spread of respiratory viruses and relieve symptoms like congestion, sore throats, and coughing. Depending on the preparation and personal tolerance, there are several dosage recommendations for ginger, which can be taken fresh, as a tea, or in powdered form.

Another vigorous antiviral plant that may help with respiratory infections and influenza is garlic (Allium sativum). Allicin, a sulfur-based molecule with antibacterial and immune-stimulating qualities, is found in garlic. Garlic has been shown in studies to decrease viral replication and boost immunological responses, which may help prevent colds and the flu. Although dosage recommendations and efficacy may differ, consuming raw garlic or supplements containing the vegetable may help support immune function and lower the risk of respiratory infections.

Herbal therapy has long employed licorice root (Glycyrrhiza glabra) to treat respiratory infections like the flu, colds, and coughs. Glycyrrhizin is found in licorice root, a substance with antiviral, anti-inflammatory, and immune-modulating properties. According to research, licorice root may lessen cough symptoms, lessen respiratory tract irritation, and stop the spread of viruses. Several types of licorice root are available, including teas, lozenges, and capsules. It should be taken carefully because it may have adverse effects or interfere with certain medications.

Apart from these herbal medicines, oregano, thyme, peppermint, and eucalyptus are also frequently used as antiviral herbs for influenza and respiratory infections. The volatile oils in oregano and thyme have antibacterial qualities that can help stop the growth of respiratory viruses and relieve symptoms like congestion and cough. Menthol, found in peppermint and eucalyptus, can be administered locally as a chest rub or inhaled as steam to help calm irritated airways and reduce nasal congestion.

When utilizing antiviral herbs for respiratory infections and influenza, it's critical to select reliable suppliers for high-quality goods and adhere to dosage guidelines found on product labels. To guarantee safety and effectiveness, speaking with a licensed healthcare provider is essential, particularly for people with underlying medical issues, expectant or nursing mothers, and kids. Antiviral herbs can provide natural relief from respiratory infections and influenza. Still, they should only be used as one component of a comprehensive sickness management strategy that includes rest, fluids, and other supportive measures. Antiviral herbs can effectively boost immune function and respiratory health with the proper care and attention, assisting in the fight against influenza and enhancing general well-being.

## Formulas and recipes for respiratory health

Comprise a broad spectrum of herbal medicines and natural preparations intended to support lung health, reduce respiratory symptoms, and enhance lung function in general. These concoctions target a range of respiratory ailments, such as colds, coughs, flu, asthma, bronchitis, and allergies, by utilizing the healing qualities of aromatic spices, nutritious foods, and medicinal herbs. You can improve respiratory health and vitality with various formulas and recipes ranging from contemporary culinary innovations to traditional herbal formulations that can be included in everyday routines.

A typical herbal remedy for respiratory health is called the "lung tonic" or "lung support" formula; it usually consists of a combination of herbs that have immune-stimulating, expectorant, and antitussive qualities. Among the common constituents included in lung tonic formulae are mullein leaf, marshmallow root, thyme, elecampane, and licorice root. These herbs can ease irritated airways, lessen coughing, assist break up mucus, and boost immunity. To relieve respiratory symptoms and support lung health, lung tonic formulae come in a variety of formats, such as teas, tinctures, capsules, and syrups. They can be used as needed.

The "cold and flu" formula is another herbal remedy traditionally used for respiratory health. Its purpose is to boost immunity and alleviate cold and flu-related symptoms. Often included in this combination are herbs like echinacea, elderberry, ginger, and garlic that have antiviral, immune-stimulating, and fever-reducing qualities. These herbs are thought to lessen the length and intensity of cold and flu symptoms, such as fever, sore throat, congestion, and body pains. Cold and flu remedies can be taken either as a prophylactic measure during the cold and flu season or as needed to relieve symptoms as soon as they appear. They come in a variety of forms, such as teas, tinctures, capsules, and syrups.

Numerous food recipes and DIY cures can enhance lung function and improve respiratory health in addition to conventional herbal solutions. A well-liked cure is honey and lemon tea, which combines the calming qualities of honey with the zesty, vitamin C-rich taste of lemon. Lemon aids in mucus thinness and offers antioxidant support, while honey is well-known for its antibacterial and calming effects on the throat. Utilizing essential oils like eucalyptus, peppermint, or tea tree oil in a steam inhalation is another do-it-yourself therapy that can help relieve respiratory symptoms, clear clogged airways, and reduce inflammation.

Combining milk's calming and warming effects with the anti-inflammatory and immune-modulating qualities of turmeric, turmeric milk, commonly referred to as "golden milk," is another well-liked treatment for respiratory health. Turmeric milk, sometimes known as "golden milk," combines the anti-inflammatory and immune-modulating properties of turmeric with the soothing and warming properties of milk to create a popular remedy for respiratory health. It may strengthen the immune system and lessen respiratory tract irritation. In addition to turmeric, other ingredients that are frequently added to turmeric milk include ginger, cinnamon, black pepper, and honey, all of which have further medicinal advantages for respiratory health.

The health of your respiratory system is further enhanced by soups and broths prepared with immune-stimulating substances like ginger, garlic, onions, and medicinal mushrooms. The body's natural defenses against respiratory infections can be bolstered by the antibacterial, anti-inflammatory, and immune-stimulating chemicals present in these substances. Spices and herbs like sage, oregano, rosemary, and thyme can be added to soups and broths to increase their antibacterial and antioxidant content and improve their respiratory effects even more.

In summary, a variety of herbal remedies and culinary creations can support lung function, lessen respiratory symptoms, and improve overall respiratory well-being. These can be found in respiratory health formulations and recipes. There are many ways to improve respiratory health and energy, ranging from conventional herbal remedies to cutting-edge culinary techniques. A person can maintain optimal respiratory health and well-being by adding these formulas and recipes into everyday routines, whether it's a nourishing soup, a calming herbal tea, or a home treatment. As usual, it's crucial to seek the advice of a licensed healthcare provider for tailored advice and suggestions based on unique health needs and situations.

# CHAPTER VI

# Herbs for Systemic Viral Infections

**Antiviral herbs for gastrointestinal viruses**

They supply organic substitutes for conventional therapies and bolster the immune system's defenses against viral infections that impact the gastrointestinal tract. Especially in susceptible groups like children, the elderly, and people with compromised immune systems, intestinal viruses, such as norovirus, rotavirus, and adenovirus, can cause symptoms like nausea, vomiting, diarrhea, abdominal pain, and fever. These symptoms can result in discomfort and potentially severe complications. Through the utilization of medicinal herbs' antiviral qualities, people can aid in preventing and relieving symptoms related to viral gastrointestinal infections.

The root ginger (Zingiber officinale), which has a long history of traditional use in treating digestive disorders, is one of the most well-known antiviral medicines for gastrointestinal viruses. Bioactive substances found in ginger, such as shogaol and gingerol, have strong antibacterial and anti-inflammatory qualities. These substances have been demonstrated to impede the growth of many viruses, such as rotavirus and norovirus, by disrupting viral replication and adjusting immune responses. Ginger may help relieve the symptoms of gastrointestinal virus infections, including nausea, vomiting, and diarrhea. It can be powdered, consumed raw, or steeped as tea.

Another herbal medicine that may have antiviral qualities against gastrointestinal viruses is peppermint (Mentha x piperita). Menthol, a substance with antibacterial and antispasmodic properties found in peppermint, helps relieve digestive discomfort and symptoms like cramping, diarrhea, and stomach pain. Studies have shown that peppermint oil can stop the growth of rotavirus and norovirus, which may be beneficial for digestive health. Oral administration of peppermint tea or diluted peppermint oil can alleviate symptoms associated with gastrointestinal viral infections.

With its antiviral and anti-inflammatory qualities, licorice root (Glycyrrhiza glabra) is a traditional herbal treatment that may help with stomach infections. Glycyrrhizin, a substance found in licorice root, has strong antiviral properties against a variety of viruses, such as rotavirus and norovirus. Licorice root is a valuable herb for treating gastrointestinal viral infection symptoms, including diarrhea and stomach pain, since it has also been demonstrated to help lower intestinal inflammation and encourage mucosal repair. For gastrointestinal assistance, licorice root tea or capsules can be used orally.

Chamomile (Matricaria chamomilla), a mild herb with calming and soothing properties on the digestive system, is another herbal treatment for gastrointestinal viruses. Bioactive substances found in chamomile include terpenoids and flavonoids, which have antibacterial, anti-inflammatory, and spasmolytic qualities. Chamomile tea can help lessen the symptoms of gastrointestinal viral infections, such as nausea, vomiting, diarrhea, and abdominal pain, in addition to promoting relaxation and relieving stress. These benefits boost the immune system and aid in the healing process.

Apart from individual herbs, herbal blends and formulations exist that are specially made to target viruses that affect the gastrointestinal tract and promote healthy digestion. Herbal teas, for instance, that combine ginger, peppermint, licorice root, and chamomile can support gastrointestinal health holistically by addressing symptoms like nausea, vomiting, diarrhea, and abdominal pain, as well as having immune-stimulating and anti-inflammatory properties. Oral use of these herbal formulations as teas or infusions is possible; dosage recommendations vary based on the particular product and the health requirements of the individual.

Antiviral herbs can provide a natural remedy for gastrointestinal viral infections. Still, it's crucial to remember that they should only be used in conjunction with other holistic methods of managing disease, such as enough rest, water, and diet. People with underlying medical issues or those experiencing severe or protracted symptoms should speak with a licensed healthcare provider for individualized advice and recommendations. In the face of viral infections affecting the digestive system, people can improve gastrointestinal health and enhance general well-being by including antiviral herbs in their daily routines.

## Herbal support for viral skin conditions

It provides a holistic, all-natural method for easing symptoms and encouraging recovery. Herpes simplex, often known as cold sores, shingles, herpes zoster, and human papillomavirus warts, are examples of viral skin disorders that can be painful, embarrassing, and cause discomfort. Herbal remedies offer alternatives to traditional treatments, which concentrate on symptom management and antiviral drugs. These treatments help reduce symptoms, boost immunity, and encourage skin healing.

Lemon balm (Melissa officinalis), a member of the mint family with antiviral solid qualities, is one of the most well-known herbal treatments for viral skin diseases. It has been shown that bioactive components of lemon balm, such as rosmarinic acid and caffeic acid, inhibit the herpes simplex virus from replicating and reduce the frequency and severity of cold sore outbreaks. Applying lemon balm cream or ointment topically can help calm cold sore lesions, lessen discomfort and inflammation, and hasten healing. Lemon balm tea can also be taken orally to boost immunity and lower the likelihood of repeated outbreaks.

Tea tree oil (Melaleuca alternifolia), an essential oil with broad-spectrum antibacterial and antiviral qualities, is another natural treatment for viral skin problems. It has been shown that terpenes in tea tree oil, such as terpinen-4-ol, inhibit the growth of the herpes simplex and human papillomavirus. Topically applying diluted tea tree oil can help minimize wart size and length, ease itching and irritation, and encourage skin healing. To prevent irritation or allergic responses, tea tree oil must be carefully diluted and tested on a patch of skin before being applied.

Another herbal medicine with anti-inflammatory, antiviral, and wound-healing qualities that may help viral skin disorders is calendula (Calendula officinalis). Flavonoids, triterpenoids, and polysaccharides found in calendula have been demonstrated to support tissue healing and lower inflammation. Calendula cream or ointment applied topically can help calm irritated skin, lessen pain and itching, and hasten the healing of lesions linked to viral skin disorders like shingles and herpes simplex. Because calendula treatments are mild and easily absorbed, even those with sensitive skin can use them.

Hypericum perforatum, sometimes known as St. John's wort, is an herbal medicine with antidepressant and anti-inflammatory qualities that has been traditionally used for viral skin problems. Hypericin and hyperforin, two bioactive substances found in St. John's wort, have antiviral properties against the varicella-zoster virus, which causes shingles, and the herpes simplex virus. St.

John's Wort oil or cream, when applied topically, can aid with shingle lesions' discomfort, inflammation, and itching while encouraging skin healing and minimizing scarring. When using St. John's wort topically, staying out of the sun is crucial as this can exacerbate photosensitivity.

Another herbal medicine with antiviral and anti-inflammatory qualities that may help with viral skin disorders is licorice root (Glycyrrhiza glabra). Glycyrrhizin, a substance found in licorice root, has been demonstrated to stop the herpes simplex virus from replicating and to lessen skin inflammation. Applying licorice root extract or gel topically can help relieve cold sore lesions, lessen discomfort and swelling, and hasten the healing process. Preparations made from licorice root are usually safe and well-tolerated, but continued use may have negative consequences, including skin irritation or systemic effects from the glycyrrhizin concentration.

Herbal blends and formulations specially made for viral skin problems are available in addition to these individual herbs. These blends and formulations combine many herbs with complementary qualities to offer complete support for skin health and healing. A combination of antiviral, anti-inflammatory, and wound-healing herbs, such as calendula, lemon balm, tea tree oil, St. John's wort, and licorice root, among others, may be included in these formulations. By using these herbal formulations topically, skin lesions linked to viral skin disorders can heal more quickly, have symptom relief, and have less viral reproduction.

Herbal treatments can provide natural relief for viral skin diseases. Still, it's vital to remember that they should only be used as a supplement to a complete skincare and general health regimen. People with underlying medical issues or severe or persistent symptoms should speak with a licensed healthcare provider for individualized advice and recommendations. In the face of viral skin diseases, people can help control symptoms, encourage healing, and preserve healthy skin by adding herbal support to their skincare routines.

## Managing systemic viral infections with herbal medicine

It involves applying medicinal herbs' healing qualities to enhance immune system function, lessen viral replication, treat symptoms, and advance general health and well-being. Human immunodeficiency virus (HIV), hepatitis viruses, and influenza are systemic viral infections that impact several organs and tissues throughout the body, resulting in a wide range of symptoms and possible problems. Herbal medicine provides natural alternatives to conventional medicines that can assist conventional therapy and strengthen the body's defenses against viral infections. In contrast, traditional treatments for systemic viral infections typically require antiviral drugs and supportive care.

Focusing on immune support is one of the main strategies for using herbal therapy to treat systemic viral infections. Herbs with well-known immune-boosting qualities, like echinacea, astragalus, and elderberry, have long been used to strengthen immunity and improve resistance to illnesses. White tea increases the generation of leukocytes, while astragalus has polysaccharides that aid in regulating the immune system. Flavonoids, which are abundant in elderberries, have been demonstrated to prevent viral replication and lessen the intensity and duration of colds and the flu. You can take these immune-boosting herbs orally as teas, tinctures, or capsules to help bolster the body's defenses against viral infections that target the system.

Antiviral herbs are essential for treating systemic viral infections as well as immune support. Strong antiviral qualities found in herbs like garlic, licorice root, and olive leaf can help prevent viral growth and lower the body's viral burden. Glycyrrhizin, a substance found in licorice root, has been demonstrated to prevent the growth of certain viruses, such as hepatitis, herpes simplex, and influenza viruses. Olive leaves contain oleeuropein, a bioactive compound that exhibits antiviral activity against a range of infections, including HIV and hepatitis. Garlic produces a substance called allicin, which has been shown to inhibit the growth of influenza, respiratory syncytial, and herpes simplex viruses. These antiviral herbs can be used orally as teas, tinctures, or supplements to treat systemic viral infections and lessen symptoms.

Herbal remedies created especially to treat systemic viral infections may incorporate a variety of herbs with complementary qualities to offer complete immune system support, antiviral action, and symptom alleviation. Herbal blends, for instance, that combine antiviral herbs like garlic, licorice root, and olive leaf with immune-supportive herbs like echinacea, astragalus, and elderberry can help boost the body's defenses, lessen viral replication, and ease symptoms of systemic viral infections. These herbal mixtures are available in various forms, including teas, tinctures, capsules, and syrups, and can be tailored to suit individual health needs and preferences.

Topical herbal medicines can be helpful in treating systemic viral infections in addition to oral medication, primarily if the virus affects the skin or mucous membranes. Herbs with antiviral, antibacterial, and wound-healing qualities, like tea tree oil, lemon balm, and calendula, can lessen the growth of viruses, calm inflamed tissues, and aid in the healing of wounds. When these herbal medicines are used topically as creams, ointments, or compresses, they can offer localized relief from the discomfort, inflammation, and itching associated with systemic viral infections that affect the skin or mucous membranes.

Herbal medication can provide natural support for treating systemic viral infections, but it should not be used in place of conventional medical therapies or medical professionals' guidance. Patients with systemic viral infections should collaborate closely with their medical professionals to create a thorough treatment plan that may incorporate unconventional and traditional medicine. Herbal medicines should also be used cautiously, particularly in those with allergies, underlying medical issues, or sensitivity to particular herbs. Herbs that support the immune system, fight viruses, and relieve symptoms can be incorporated into treatment plans to help people manage systemic viral infections and enhance their general health and well-being.

# CHAPTER VII

# Herbal Allies for Specific Viruses

## Herbs for herpes simplex virus (HSV)

Provide natural substitutes for controlling outbreaks, reducing symptoms, and boosting immunity in those afflicted with this widespread viral infection. Herpes simplex virus (HSV), in particular types 1 and 2, can cause painful, recurrent lesions on the lips, genitalia, and other mucosal membranes, causing discomfort, stigma, and emotional suffering. Herbal medicines offer more options for people looking for holistic approaches to controlling their health, even while traditional therapies like antiviral pharmaceuticals can help lessen the frequency and intensity of outbreaks.

Lemon balm (Melissa officinalis), a member of the mint family renowned for its antiviral and calming qualities, is one of the herbs for HSV that has been investigated the most. It has been shown that bioactive components of lemon balm, such as rosmarinic acid and caffeic acid, inhibit HSV replication and reduce the frequency and duration of cold sore outbreaks. Topically, lemon balm cream or ointment can help calm sores, lessen discomfort and inflammation, and encourage quicker healing. Lemon balm tea can also be taken orally to boost immunity and lower the likelihood of repeated outbreaks.

Glycyrrhizin, an antiviral and immune-modulating component found in licorice root (Glycyrrhiza glabra), is another plant that may be beneficial for HSV. It has been demonstrated that glycyrrhizin inhibits HSV replication and lowers inflammation in the afflicted area. Applying licorice root extract or gel topically can help reduce HSV lesion-related discomfort, itching, and burning. Moreover, licorice root can be taken orally as a supplement or tea to boost immunity and lessen the frequency of breakouts.

Another herb that's frequently used for viral infections, like HSV, and immune support is echinacea (Echinacea purpurea). White blood cell production is stimulated by echinacea, which also strengthens the body's defenses against viral illnesses. Although there is no data on how specifically echinacea affects HSV, several studies have indicated that taking echinacea orally at the first sign of symptoms may help lessen the frequency and intensity of cold sore outbreaks. Echinacea products, such as teas, tinctures, and capsules, can be utilized as a component of a complete strategy to improve immune function and manage HSV outbreaks.

Bees gather propolis, a sticky material, from tree buds and sap, and it has also demonstrated promise in the management of HSV. Bioactive substances found in propolis include phenolic acids and flavonoids, which have immune-modulating and antiviral qualities. Research has indicated that using propolis extracts topically in afflicted areas can prevent HSV proliferation and decrease the frequency of outbreaks. For those with HSV, propolis lotions or ointments may help calm lesions, lessen discomfort and inflammation, and encourage quicker healing.

Herbal formulations and blends created especially for HSV are also available in addition to these individual herbs. These blends and formulations combine many herbs with complementary qualities to offer complete support for immune function, antiviral activity, and symptom relief. Herbal mixtures that contain licorice root, propolis, echinacea, and lemon balm, for instance, can help boost the immune system, lessen viral replication, and ease the symptoms of HSV outbreaks. These herbal concoctions can be customized to meet specific health needs and preferences and come in a variety of formats, such as lotions, ointments, tinctures, and capsules.

It is crucial to remember that although herbal medicines might provide HSV outbreaks with a natural solution, they shouldn't take the place of traditional medical treatments or medical professionals' guidance. Patients with HSV should collaborate closely with their medical professionals to create a thorough treatment plan that might incorporate unconventional and traditional medications. Herbal medicines should also be used cautiously, particularly in those with allergies, underlying medical issues, or sensitivity to particular herbs. People with HSV can improve their overall health and well-being and better control outbreaks by adding immune-supportive, antiviral, and symptom-relieving herbs to their treatment regimens.

## Antiviral herbs for human papillomavirus (HPV)

Provide natural remedies for immune system support, HPV infection management, and possible reduction of consequences, including genital warts and cervical cancer. Sexually transmitted HPV infection is widespread and can lead to several health problems, such as warts on the genitalia and several cancers, including cervical cancer. Herbal medicines are gaining popularity as a potential means of managing HPV infections and promoting general health, even though vaccines are now available to prevent some strains of the virus.

Green tea (Camellia sinensis), which includes bioactive compounds like catechins, especially epigallocatechin gallate (EGCG), which is renowned for its antiviral and antioxidant effects, is one of the herbs for HPV that has been investigated the most. Research has demonstrated that EGCG can prevent HPV replication and lower the chance that cervical cancer will advance. Green tea extract or ointment applied topically may help lessen the size and severity of genital warts brought on by HPV infections. Regular use of green tea may enhance immune system performance and lower the risk of HPV infections.

Echinacea, or Echinacea purpurea, is another herb that may help with HPV. It has been used traditionally to treat viral infections and boost the immune system. White blood cell production is stimulated by echinacea, which also strengthens the body's defenses against viral infections, including HPV. Although echinacea's precise effects on HPV are still poorly understood, some studies have indicated that echinacea may be able to lessen the frequency and severity of genital warts brought on by HPV infections. Echinacea formulations, such as tinctures, capsules, and teas, can be utilized as a complete strategy to enhance immune system performance and manage HPV infections.

Another herb with possible antiviral qualities that may help people with HPV infections is turmeric (Curcuma longa). Turmeric's key ingredient, curcumin, has been demonstrated to have antiviral properties against a number of viruses, including HPV. Additionally, turmeric possesses anti-inflammatory and antioxidant properties that may help reduce inflammation and oxidative stress related to HPV infections. Although there is little information particularly linking turmeric to HPV, adding turmeric to food or taking supplements may boost immunity and lower the chance of problems from HPV.

Strong antiviral properties found in garlic (Allium sativum) may also help those with HPV infections. Allicin, a substance found in garlic, has immune-stimulating and broad-spectrum antibacterial qualities. Research has demonstrated that garlic extract can lower the risk of cervical cancer progression and limit the replication of a number of viruses, including HPV. Regularly consuming raw garlic or supplements containing garlic may boost immune system performance and lower the risk of problems from HPV.

Herbal formulations and blends created especially for HPV infections are also available in addition to these individual herbs. These blends and formulations combine many herbs with complementary qualities to offer complete support for immune function, antiviral activity, and symptom relief. Herbal mixtures, including garlic, echinacea, turmeric, and green tea extract, may boost immunity, stop the spread of viruses, and lower the risk of HPV-related disorders like cervical cancer and genital warts. These herbal mixtures are available in a variety of forms, including teas, tinctures, and capsules, and can be tailored to match individual health needs and tastes.

Herbal medicines can provide natural assistance for HPV infections, but they shouldn't take the place of traditional medical treatments or medical professionals' guidance. Patients with HPV should collaborate closely with their medical professionals to create a thorough treatment strategy that might incorporate alternative and traditional medications. Herbal medicines should also be used cautiously, particularly in those with allergies, underlying medical issues, or sensitivity to particular herbs. Individuals with HPV can improve their overall health and well-being and help control infections more effectively by adding immune-supportive, antiviral, and symptom-relieving herbs to their treatment regimens.


## Herbal remedies for hepatitis viruses

Hepatitis viruses, specifically hepatitis B (HBV) and hepatitis C (HCV), pose a severe threat to global health, impacting millions of individuals around the globe. These viruses have the ability to inflame the liver, that may result in a variety of symptoms as well as potentially dangerous side effects like liver cancer and cirrhosis. Even while supportive care and antiviral medications are still frequently used treatments for hepatitis viruses, herbal therapies are gaining popularity as complementary or alternative approaches. For those infected with hepatitis viruses, herbal medicines provide natural components that may help improve liver function, reduce inflammation, and suppress viral reproduction.

Milk thistle (Silybum marianum) is one of the herbs for hepatitis viruses that have been investigated the most. A class of bioactive substances called silymarin, found in milk thistle, has hepatoprotective solid effects. Given its demonstrated antiviral, anti-inflammatory, and antioxidant properties, silymarin is a highly effective herbal treatment for hepatitis virus infections and liver health issues. Research has indicated that in patients with hepatitis B and hepatitis C infections, milk thistle extract can help lower liver inflammation, enhance liver function tests, and prevent viral replication. Furthermore, milk thistle may lessen the risk of hepatocellular carcinoma and liver cirrhosis by shielding the liver from oxidative stress and pollutants.

Glycyrrhiza glabra, or licorice root, is another herbal therapy that may be beneficial for hepatitis viruses. Glycyrrhizin, a substance found in licorice root, has antiviral and anti-inflammatory qualities. Preclinical research has demonstrated that glycyrrhizin reduces liver inflammation and inhibits the replication of the hepatitis B and hepatitis C viruses. Furthermore, licorice root has the potential to lessen the harm that viral infections bring to the liver by supporting liver function and encouraging liver cell regeneration. But it's crucial to remember that licorice root should only be used sparingly because overindulging might have adverse effects, including electrolyte imbalances and hypertension.

Another herbal medicine that has been traditionally used for liver health and may be beneficial for hepatitis viruses is Schisandra (Schisandra chinensis). Lignans and other bioactive substances with hepatoprotective, antioxidant, and anti-inflammatory qualities are found in Schisandra. According to preclinical research, Schisandra extract can lessen fibrosis and inflammation of the liver in animal models of hepatitis B and hepatitis C diseases. Schisandra may also help improve liver function and symptoms of viral hepatitis, including fatigue and stomach discomfort. To fully comprehend the modes of action and possible therapeutic advantages of Schisandra for hepatitis viruses, more investigation is required.

Another herb with potent anti-inflammatory and antioxidant qualities that may promote liver health and fight hepatitis viruses is turmeric (Curcuma longa). Preclinical research has demonstrated that curcumin, the key ingredient in turmeric, inhibits viral replication and reduces inflammation in the liver. Turmeric may also lessen the risk of liver damage and the advancement of hepatitis B and hepatitis C infections by shielding the liver from oxidative stress and toxins. For those with viral hepatitis, adding turmeric to their diet or taking supplements may enhance liver function and improve general health.

Herbal formulations and blends especially made for hepatitis viruses are available in addition to these individual herbs. These blends and formulations combine many herbs with complementary qualities to offer complete support for liver health and viral suppression. For example, in people with hepatitis B and hepatitis C infections, herbal blends comprising a combination of milk thistle, licorice root, schisandra, and turmeric may help strengthen the liver, reduce inflammation, and suppress viral reproduction. These herbal mixtures are available in a range of forms, including teas, tinctures, and capsules, and can be tailored to match individual health needs and tastes.

While herbal remedies can provide natural support for hepatitis viruses, it is crucial to remember that they should not be used in place of conventional medical treatments or medical advice from professionals. Patients with viral hepatitis should collaborate closely with their medical professionals to create a thorough treatment plan that may incorporate unconventional and traditional medicine. Furthermore, as herbal medicines have the potential to interfere with some pharmaceuticals or have adverse effects, they should be taken with caution, particularly in people with underlying medical disorders or those on medication. Hepatitis virus patients can enhance liver function and general well-being by adding immune-supportive, anti-inflammatory, and hepatoprotective herbs to their treatment regimens.

# CHAPTER VIII

# Integrating Herbal Medicine with Conventional Treatments

## Understanding potential interactions between herbs and medications

It is essential to guarantee the secure and efficient treatment of medical disorders. For millennia, traditional medical systems have employed herbs as a means of promoting health and treating a range of diseases. Herbs can, however, interact with some prescriptions in ways that could reduce their efficacy, raise the possibility of adverse side effects, or even result in life-threatening health issues. Herbs can affect how the body reacts to pharmaceuticals through various mechanisms, including changes in drug metabolism, absorption, distribution, and excretion. Another type of interaction is called pharmacodynamic interaction.

Herb-drug interactions primarily stem from the alteration of liver-resident drug-metabolizing enzymes, specifically cytochrome P450 (CYP) enzymes. Bioactive chemicals found in many herbs have the ability to either activate or inhibit these enzymes, changing how drugs are metabolized and how much of them are in the blood. For instance, it is known that St. John's wort (Hypericum perforatum) induces CYP3A4 and other CYP enzymes, which can lead to a drop in the blood levels of several drugs, such as oral contraceptives, antidepressants, and antiretrovirals. On the other hand, substances in grapefruit juice inhibit CYP3A4, which raises blood levels of drugs that this enzyme metabolizes, including immunosuppressants, statins, and calcium channel blockers.

Herbs can influence medication absorption, distribution, and excretion through a variety of ways, in addition to interactions mediated by enzymes. Certain herbs, for example, have the ability to improve the absorption of medications by modifying intestinal permeability or enhancing gastrointestinal motility. This might result in increased drug levels in the blood and raise the possibility of toxicity. On the other hand, some herbs have the potential to impede drug absorption through the formation of complexes with pharmaceuticals in the gastrointestinal tract or by vying for absorption sites, thus decreasing the drug's effectiveness and bioavailability.

Additionally, herbs have the ability to modify tissue permeability or bind to plasma proteins, which can change how pharmaceuticals are distributed throughout the body and affect both the safety and efficacy of medications.

Also, herbs and pharmaceuticals may interact pharmacodynamically, meaning that when taken together, the body may experience antagonistic, synergistic, or additive effects. For instance, sedative plants like kava or valerian root may intensify the effects of sedative drugs, causing respiratory depression or excessive drowsiness. Similarly, taking blood-thinning drugs like aspirin or warfarin along with plants that have anticoagulant qualities, like garlic or ginkgo biloba, may make bleeding more likely. On the other hand, herbs like green tea or turmeric that have anti-inflammatory or antioxidant qualities can either lessen the adverse effects of some drugs on the body or increase their beneficial effects.

Healthcare professionals should ask patients about their medications, including over-the-counter drugs, dietary supplements, and herbal therapies, to reduce the possibility of herb-drug interactions. It is important to encourage patients to reveal all the herbal products they take, together with the dosage, frequency, and length of usage. Healthcare professionals should also advise patients on how to reduce the possibility of drug interactions and inform them of the advantages and possible risks of using herbs along with prescriptions.

Before beginning or stopping any herbal medicines, patients should also be urged to speak with a skilled healthcare provider, such as a pharmacist or herbalist, especially if they are taking a prescription for severe or chronic health concerns. Based on the patient's medical history, current prescriptions, and specific herb-drug interactions reported in the literature, healthcare providers can assist in assessing the possibility of herb-drug interactions. They can also offer advice on how to take herbal remedies safely and effectively, including when to take them, how much to take, and how to keep an eye out for any adverse effects or ineffectiveness.

Patients should also exercise caution when buying herbal remedies because there can be significant differences in terms of quality, strength, and purity between various brands and producers. Selecting trustworthy brands that follow sound manufacturing principles (GMP) and have undergone independent quality testing for potency and purity is advised. Additionally, consumers should be on the lookout for deceptive or unsupported claims made by producers. They should speak with medical professionals prior to utilizing any herbal products, especially those that are advertised as having therapeutic benefits or are intended to treat particular medical issues.

In conclusion, in order to ensure the safe and efficient use of both pharmaceutical treatments and herbal therapies, it is imperative to comprehend potential interactions between herbs and prescriptions. Healthcare providers and patients alike ought to be aware of the mechanisms underlying herb-drug interactions and take the necessary precautions to reduce the risk of harmful effects or ineffectiveness. Patients and healthcare providers must communicate openly to optimize patient outcomes and detect and handle potential herb-drug interactions. Healthcare practitioners can help ensure the safe and proper use of herbal medicines in conjunction with conventional pharmaceuticals by adopting evidence-based procedures for herb-drug interactions and by managing medications proactively.

## Guidelines for combining herbal and pharmaceutical approaches

Combining pharmaceutical and herbal medicine has become popular as more individuals look for integrative and holistic answers to their medical issues. Although there are many advantages to this method, there are also some drawbacks, such as herb-drug combinations and safety issues. Establishing guidelines for combining pharmaceutical and herbal treatments is necessary to guarantee the effective and safe treatment of medical conditions. These recommendations cover patient education, communication between healthcare providers and patients, concern for each patient, interaction monitoring, and evidence-based decision-making.

Patient education is the most crucial factor in safely integrating herbal and pharmacological methods into treatment. Patients must be aware of the advantages and possible risks of receiving both kinds of treatment simultaneously. This entails being aware of potential interactions between pharmaceutical medications and herbal medicines, comprehending the potential interactions between these substances, and being able to recognize and report any adverse effects or symptom changes. To enable thorough treatment planning and monitoring, patient education should also cover the significance of telling their healthcare professionals about all herbal items and pharmaceuticals they are taking.

The successful integration of herbal and pharmaceutical approaches is contingent upon effective communication between healthcare providers and patients. Patients who utilize herbal medicines and other complementary therapies should feel comfortable discussing them with healthcare providers in a supportive and nonjudgmental atmosphere. Encouraging patients to express their worries, pose inquiries, and participate actively in the healthcare decision-making process is crucial. Thanks to this collaborative approach, improved patient satisfaction and treatment adherence can result from treatment regimens customized to each patient's unique needs and preferences.

When integrating herbal and pharmacological methods into healthcare, healthcare providers should consider unique patient variables in addition to patient education and communication. Age, gender, medical history, past drug use, and lifestyle choices are some of the variables that can affect the likelihood of herb-drug interactions as well as how well treatment plans work. Patients with certain medical conditions or those taking several medications may need more frequent monitoring and customized treatment strategies to reduce the risk of side effects and maximize treatment success. Healthcare professionals should also be aware of patient's cultural and personal views about healthcare and consider these when designing a treatment plan.

When combining herbal and pharmaceutical methods in healthcare, it is critical to watch for herb-drug interactions and therapeutic efficacy. To detect any possible interactions or therapeutic failures, healthcare professionals should routinely evaluate patients for indications of side effects, alterations in symptoms, and response to treatment. This could entail regularly performing physical examinations, laboratory testing, and symptom evaluations. In order to enable rapid intervention and necessary treatment plan adjustments, patients should be urged to report any new symptoms or changes in their health status to their healthcare professionals as soon as possible.

A further essential component of integrating herbal and pharmacological methods into healthcare is evidence-based decision-making. Healthcare professionals should be current on the most recent findings and clinical recommendations on herbal medicines, integrative healthcare procedures, and interactions between herbs and drugs. This could entail reading peer-reviewed publications, attending continuing education seminars, and speaking with integrative medicine specialists. Healthcare professionals can make well-informed decisions emphasizing patient safety and maximizing treatment results by incorporating evidence-based practices into treatment planning.

Additionally, when combining herbal and pharmaceutical approaches to healing, healthcare providers should be vigilant in addressing possible interactions between herbs and drugs and safety concerns. During patient consultations and medication reconciliation procedures, this may entail performing thorough medication reviews, including those involving herbal products. In order to promote coordinated and comprehensive care, healthcare practitioners should also teach patients the value of disclosing information about their use of herbal medicines and other complementary therapies to all members of their healthcare team, including pharmacists and specialists.

In summary, recommendations for integrating pharmaceutical and herbal medicine are critical to guaranteeing the secure and efficient treatment of medical diseases. These recommendations cover patient education, communication between healthcare providers and patients, concern for each patient, interaction monitoring, and evidence-based decision-making. By adhering to these recommendations, medical professionals can reduce the possibility of herb-drug interactions, improve treatment results, and offer patient- centered, comprehensive care that considers each patient's particular requirements and preferences.

## Case studies illustrating successful integration of herbal medicine

Herbal medicine has recently been incorporated into conventional healthcare procedures due to the growing recognition of the therapeutic value of medicinal plants and the demand for all-encompassing, customized approaches to health and wellness. Case studies show the effectiveness, safety, and clinical utility of botanical treatments in a variety of clinical contexts, offering insightful information about the successful integration of herbal medicine into patient care. This section examines several case studies demonstrating the effective incorporation of herbal medicine into medical practice, highlighting the various uses and advantages of herbal therapy for patients.

Herbal Analgesics for Chronic Pain Management Mrs. A, a 55-year-old lady, arrived with persistent lower back discomfort that was unresponsive to traditional pain relief techniques. With few options and worries about long-term opiate addiction, Mrs. A saw a naturopathic doctor, who suggested a customized herbal pain treatment regimen. The regimen comprised nerve-calming herbs like passionflower and valerian along with anti-inflammatory and analgesic herbs, including devil's claw, turmeric, ginger, and boswellia. After receiving herbal treatment for many weeks, Mrs. A reported a considerable improvement in her quality of life and pain levels. She also noted reduced dependency on prescription pain drugs and increased mobility and function.

Herbal Therapies as Supportive Care for Cancer Patients
Mr. B, a 65-year-old man, was suffering from severe side effects such as nausea, exhaustion, and appetite loss from chemotherapy for metastatic lung cancer. Mr. B sought further assistance from an integrative oncologist, who suggested an individualized herbal regimen to go along with his traditional cancer treatment. Herbs like astragalus and echinacea for immune support, ginger and peppermint for nausea treatment, and adaptogenic herbs like Rhodiola and ashwagandha for fatigue management were also part of the protocol. Mr. B was able to continue his cancer treatment with more ease and confidence after the addition of herbal medicines to his treatment plan. He reported improved symptom control, an improved quality of life, and better tolerance to chemotherapy.

Handling Digestive Issues with Herbal Treatments
Irritable bowel syndrome (IBS) symptoms, such as bloating, irregular bowel movements, and abdominal pain, were reported by 40-year-old Ms. C. Ms. C sought the advice of a holistic nutritionist to address her digestive troubles after being dissatisfied with traditional treatment choices. The nutritionist suggested dietary alterations and herbal therapies. Herbs like marshmallow root and slippery elm for mucosal protection and healing and peppermint, chamomile, and fennel for relieving gastrointestinal pain were part of the herbal treatment. Ms. C's IBS symptoms were significantly relieved with the combination of herbal therapy and dietary modifications, which improved her digestion, decreased her bloating, and enhanced her general gastrointestinal health.

Using Herbal Medicines to Treat Depression and Anxiety
Mr. D, a thirty-year-old man, was experiencing depressive and anxious symptoms, such as constant worry, poor mood, and trouble falling asleep. Mr. D sought out a

holistic psychiatrist due to concerns over the adverse effects of traditional antidepressant prescriptions. The psychiatrist suggested a complete treatment plan that included herbal medicines, psychotherapy, and lifestyle modifications. Herbs for mood support and relaxation, such as St. John's wort, lemon balm, and passionflower, as well as adaptogens for stress resilience, like rhodiola and ashwagandha, were included in the herbal protocol. Mr. D's mood, sleep, and general well-being improved with the combination of herbal therapies and holistic interventions; this allowed him to better manage his anxiety and depression without the need for medication.

With mounting proof of the effectiveness and safety of herbal medicines, incorporating herbal medicine into traditional healthcare procedures has been more and more recognized in recent years. Case studies emphasize the potential advantages of fusing conventional and contemporary treatment modalities and offer insightful information on the effective integration of herbal medicine into patient care. A number of case studies that demonstrate the effective incorporation of herbal medicine in many clinical contexts and medical disorders are included in this section.

**Herbal Medicine for Chronic Pain Management: A**
45-year-old female patient named Patient A first complained of persistent lower back discomfort brought on by a herniated lumbar disc. Even with typical interventions including physical therapy and nonsteroidal anti-inflammatory medicines (NSAIDs), the patient never fully recovered from the chronic pain and functional impairment. The patient was administered an herbal formulation with anti-inflammatory and analgesic characteristics, such as turmeric, ginger, and boswellia, as a complementary treatment to traditional medicine. Following four weeks of therapy, the patient reported a

marked improvement in her mobility and pain level, making it easier to get back to her regular activities. By adding herbal medicine, conventional therapy received additional support that improved pain management and the patient's quality of life.

Herbal Medicine for the Treatment of Insomnia The 35-year-old male patient B had a history of persistent insomnia, which was manifested by trouble falling asleep and numerous awakenings during the night. The patient's sleep difficulties persisted despite lifestyle changes and cognitive-behavioral therapy for insomnia (CBT-I), which resulted in exhaustion and poor functioning during the day. The patient was also prescribed a herbal tea blend that included chamomile, passionflower, and valerian root, all of which have soothing and anxiolytic qualities, in addition to CBT-I. The patient reported improvements in sleep length and quality, as well as a decrease in daytime tiredness and fewer nighttime awakenings, following two weeks of herbal medication. Herbal medicine integration offers a secure and efficient supplementary treatment alternative for treating insomnia and encouraging sound sleep.

Herbal Medicine as Supportive Care for Cancer Patients After receiving a breast cancer diagnosis, 55-year-old Patient C had surgery, adjuvant chemotherapy, and radiation therapy. The patient's quality of life was negatively impacted by severe side effects, such as fatigue, neuropathy, and nausea, even after receiving routine oncologic therapy. The patient was administered an herbal supplement, including peppermint, turmeric, and ginger, as part of an all-encompassing supportive care strategy. These herbs are known for their analgesic, antiemetic, and antiemetic qualities. The herbal supplement reduced the nausea and vomiting brought on by chemotherapy, eased neuropathic pain, and enhanced general health, all of which allowed the patient to undergo cancer treatment with more comfort and fortitude. The patient's treatment outcomes were optimized, and symptom management was improved by incorporating herbal medication into supportive care.

Handling Digestive Issues with Herbal Remedies The 30-year-old male patient D initially showed signs of irritable bowel syndrome (IBS), such as bloating, diarrhea, and constipation that alternated. The patient's recurring gastrointestinal issues persisted despite dietary changes and over-the-counter drugs, which had an impact on his everyday activities and productivity. The patient was recommended an herbal formulation containing peppermint, fennel, and ginger, which are known for their carminative and antispasmodic qualities and lifestyle modifications. Following a six-week herbal therapy regimen, the patient reported a decrease in symptoms associated with IBS, such as lessened abdominal pain and better bowel habits. The use of herbal medicine offered a successful and palatable therapeutic approach for gastrointestinal health improvement and the management of digestive diseases.

These case studies demonstrate the effective incorporation of herbal medicine into patient care for a variety of clinical diseases, including mental health issues, digestive issues, cancer support, and chronic pain.

Healthcare practitioners may provide patients with safe, efficient, and customized alternatives for maintaining their health and wellness by integrating herbal therapies into all-encompassing treatment regimens. Herbal medicine still has a significant role to play in helping patients of all ages and backgrounds achieve maximum health and recovery, especially in light of the growing interest in holistic and integrative approaches to healthcare.

Finally, case studies show how herbal medicine can be successfully incorporated into patient care and highlight its potential advantages in a range of clinical settings.

Healthcare professionals can provide patients with a comprehensive and individualized approach to recovery by integrating traditional herbal medicines with mainstream therapies. This supports health and well-being by addressing the root causes of illness. More research and clinical studies are required to clarify the mechanisms of action and maximize the use of herbal medicine in clinical practice as interest in integrative medicine grows.

# CHAPTER IX

# Herbal Safety and Quality Assurance

## Ensuring the safety of herbal preparations

Growing interest in holistic healthcare and natural cures has led to a spike in the use of herbal products as alternative or supplemental medications in recent years. Despite the potential therapeutic benefits of herbal products, there are still many unknowns when it comes to their safety. These include variations in plant composition, possible interactions with conventional pharmaceuticals, and the absence of defined regulatory frameworks. Comprehensive strategies that cover sourcing, manufacture, distribution, regulation, and consumer education must be implemented across the whole lifetime of herbal medicines to address these issues and protect public health.

The purity and integrity of the basic botanical materials are the primary determinants of the safety of herbal remedies. Since an excellent range of plant species is used in herbal medicine, it is crucial to accurately identify and authenticate botanical substances to avoid contamination, adulteration, or mislabeling. A number of methods are used to confirm the identification and purity of plant materials, including chemical profiling, DNA barcoding, and macroscopic and microscopic inspection. Strict testing procedures are also used to check for any impurities, including pesticides, heavy metals, microbiological diseases, and hazardous substances, guaranteeing that herbal remedies satisfy high-quality requirements and present the least risk to customers.

Standardized production techniques and quality control measures at the ingredient level are essential for guaranteeing the uniformity and safety of herbal products. To preserve hygienic conditions, avoid cross-contamination, and guarantee precise dosing and consistency of product formulations, good manufacturing practices, or GMPs, are essential. Following established SOPs (standard operating protocols) helps decrease variability between batches and guarantees that herbal products are manufactured under controlled settings that prioritize safety and efficacy, from harvesting and extraction to formulation and packing.

Moreover, regulatory supervision is essential to offer a structure for evaluating herbal remedies' efficacy, safety, and quality. The necessity for standardized standards and open regulatory procedures is becoming more widely acknowledged, even though regulatory techniques differ significantly between nations and regions in order to safeguard the public's health and ease the entry of herbal goods onto the market. Regulatory agencies are crucial in assessing scientific data, establishing labeling specifications, setting safety thresholds for pollutants, and monitoring compliance with regulatory standards via audits, inspections, and post-market surveillance systems.

Initiatives aimed at educating and raising consumer awareness are crucial in addition to regulatory actions to encourage responsible and well-informed usage of herbal remedies. A large number of customers may be ignorant of the possible risks connected to herbal products, such as interactions with prescription drugs, contraindications for specific populations, and the necessity of speaking with medical specialists before beginning herbal therapy. By giving customers access to precise and lucid information regarding herbal remedies' advantages, drawbacks, and restrictions, they are better equipped to make decisions that put their health and well-being first.

The ongoing attempts to ensure the safety of herbal preparations continue to meet obstacles, particularly in the context of international trade, where products may originate from multiple regions with varying regulatory requirements and quality standards. Collaborative initiatives are required to address these issues, including public and private sector stakeholders, academia, and the healthcare business. A few examples of what this might entail are efforts to strengthen quality control capabilities, harmonize regulatory frameworks, enhance post-market surveillance systems, and encourage research on the efficacy and safety of herbal treatments.

To sum up, safeguarding the security of herbal remedies necessitates a comprehensive strategy that incorporates regulatory supervision, standardized production procedures, quality control methods, and consumer education initiatives. Stakeholders can protect the public's health while maximizing the therapeutic benefits of botanical medicine, reducing potential hazards, and boosting public confidence in herbal medicines by addressing these issues comprehensively. To maximize the potential benefits of herbal preparations for global healthcare systems, safety and quality must be given top priority in their research, regulation, and use, given the growing popularity of natural treatments.

## Quality control measures for herbal products

Recently, herbal products have become extremely popular because of their perceived naturalness and possible health advantages. It is difficult to ensure the quality and safety of these goods due to the complexity of the production processes and the unpredictable nature of plant-based components. To satisfy these requirements, stringent quality control measures are required at every stage of the production process, from acquiring raw materials to distributing the final product.

Identifying and authenticating botanical substances is a critical component of quality control for herbal products. This entails confirming the authenticity of plant materials using various techniques, including chemical analysis, DNA testing, and microscopic and macroscopic inspections. By recognizing botanicals, manufacturers can lower the danger of adulteration or contamination and ensure that the right plant species are used.

Ensuring the quality and purity of the botanical substances becomes crucial after they have been verified. In this context, testing for pesticides, heavy metals, microbiological contamination, and other potentially hazardous materials are examples of quality control procedures. Herbal extracts' chemical composition and purity are frequently evaluated through the use of analytical procedures such as thin-layer chromatography (TLC), gas chromatography-mass spectrometry (GC-MS), and high-performance liquid chromatography (HPLC).

Physical and organoleptic evaluations are significant components of quality control for herbal products, in addition to chemical analysis. These tests look at things like flavor, texture, color, and odor to ensure everything is consistent and up to predetermined standards of quality. Any departure from these benchmarks could indicate problems with the raw ingredients or the manufacturing process.

Standard operating protocols (SOPs), which should be devised and adhered to strictly at every production stage, including harvesting, extraction, formulation, and packaging, are another essential component of quality control for herbal products. This reduces variances between batches and aids in maintaining consistency in product quality.

In addition, it is imperative to employ reasonable manufacturing procedures (GMP) to guarantee the hygienic production of herbal products while adhering to regulatory standards. This includes keeping facilities and equipment clean, providing workers with sufficient training, and keeping track of all production activities—regulatory bodies' routine audits and inspections aid in ensuring that GMP guidelines are followed.

Herbal items must also be stored, transported, and distributed to maintain quality control. Proper storage conditions—such as controlled temperature and humidity—are crucial to stop deterioration and preserve product stability. Thorough labeling and packaging practices also help protect herbal products from external contaminants and ensure that consumers are given correct product information.

Finally, continuous observation and assessment are essential to herbal product quality control. Feedback from customers and medical professionals, in addition to regular testing and item analysis, provide crucial information on the effectiveness and caliber of products. Initiatives for continuous improvement based on these findings encourage innovation and raise industry standards for quality in the herbal goods sector.

In conclusion, thorough quality control procedures must be implemented throughout the production chain to guarantee the quality and safety of herbal products. Every stage of the production process, from standardizing manufacturing procedures and stringent testing protocols to authenticating and identifying botanical ingredients, is essential to providing consumers with high-quality herbal goods. Manufacturers may increase consumer confidence in their goods and support the market's ongoing expansion for herbal products by following these guidelines and legal criteria.

## Potential risks and side effects of herbal antivirals

In recent years, there has been a considerable increase in interest in studying herbal antivirals as substitute medicinal agents, especially in light of the shortcomings of traditional antiviral drugs and the emergence of new infectious illnesses. Herbal treatments have a lot of promise in the fight against viral infections, but it's essential to understand that hazards are involved. To achieve safe and effective treatment outcomes, the use of herbal antivirals carries several possible hazards and side effects that need to be carefully considered and handled. A thorough analysis of the pharmacological characteristics, safety profiles, and possible interactions between herbal antivirals and conventional drugs, as well as physiological processes, is necessary to comprehend these dangers.

The intricacy and diversity of their pharmacology are one of the main dangers connected to herbal antivirals. Herbal treatments, in contrast to pharmaceutical drugs, which usually include only one active ingredient, frequently have many bioactive components that can have antagonistic or synergistic effects on the body. Because of their complexity, it is difficult to predict the exact pharmacokinetics and pharmacodynamics of herbal antivirals, which raises the risk of side effects and increases the variability of treatment results. Further complicating herbal remedies' safety and efficacy profiles are the considerable variations in quality and potency resulting from plant species, growing circumstances, harvesting methods, and processing procedures.

Using natural antivirals carries a serious risk of negative reactions and side effects. Herbal medicines can have negative consequences ranging from slight stomach discomfort to severe allergic reactions or organ poisoning, despite the fact that they are frequently thought of as natural and intrinsically safe. As an illustration, plants like

St. When used in excessive dosages or over extended periods, licorice root (Glycyrrhiza glabra), and John's wort (Hypericum perforatum) have been linked to hormone imbalances, gastrointestinal disorders, and allergic dermatitis. Similarly, in sensitive individuals, antiviral herbs like elderberry (Sambucus nigra) and echinacea (Echinacea purpurea) may aggravate autoimmune diseases or cause allergic reactions.

Moreover, people who use herbal antivirals together with conventional drugs should be very concerned about the possibility of herb-drug interactions. Compounds in many herbs can interact with the body's transporters, receptors, or enzymes that metabolize medications, changing the pharmacokinetics and effectiveness of drugs taken together. Herbs such as ginkgo (Ginkgo biloba) and garlic (Allium sativum) have been demonstrated to block cytochrome enzymes, which are essential for the metabolism of many pharmaceuticals, including antiviral treatments. Regular monitoring and caution are necessary when combining herbal and pharmaceutical therapy to avoid inferior therapeutic outcomes, increased risk of unwanted effects, or diminished pharmacological efficacy.

Furthermore, one significant safety risk related to several herbal antivirals is the possibility of herb-induced hepatotoxicity and nephrotoxicity. When taken in excess or by those who are susceptible, several herbs that are frequently used for their antiviral qualities, including green tea (Camellia sinensis), turmeric (Curcuma longa), and silymarin (derived from milk thistle, Silybum marianum), have been linked to cases of liver damage or renal dysfunction. Immune-mediated responses, idiosyncratic responses, or direct hepatotoxic or nephrotoxic effects of bioactive constituents may cause herb-induced organ toxicity. This highlights the importance of closely monitoring liver and kidney function in patients taking herbal antivirals for extended periods or at high doses.

Herbal antivirals have several safety risks and adverse effects, which are exacerbated by worries about adulteration, contamination, and mislabeling of the herbs. Research has demonstrated that herbal items may contain heavy metals, pesticides, microbiological infections, or unreported pharmaceutical medications, all of which pose serious health concerns to consumers. Moreover, the safety and effectiveness of herbal remedies may be compromised by incorrect identification or substitution of botanical constituents, which may expose users unintentionally to allergies or harmful substances. To reduce these hazards and safeguard the public's health, it is crucial to guarantee herbal antivirals' quality, authenticity, and purity by strict regulatory oversight, standardized production procedures, and quality control methods.

In summary, although herbal antivirals are a promising alternative treatment option for treating viral infections, it is essential to understand and manage their possible dangers and adverse effects. The use of herbal remedies requires evidence-based practice, careful decision-making, and close monitoring due to pharmacological complexity, variability in product quality, potential for adverse reactions and herb-drug interactions, and concerns about organ toxicity, adulteration, and contamination. Collaboration amongst manufacturers, consumers, regulatory agencies, and healthcare experts can help prioritize patient safety and well-being while navigating the complicated world of herbal medicine and realizing its therapeutic potential.

# CHAPTER X

# Herbal Antiviral Protocols

## Step-by-step protocols for addressing specific viral infections

In the field of medicine, treating viral infections requires careful procedures that are adapted to the unique characteristics of each virus. These protocols consist of systematic procedures intended to successfully identify, treat, and stop the spread of viral infections. Comprehending the distinct attributes of various viruses is crucial for formulating focused approaches to alleviate their consequences. The influenza virus is one such virus that has attracted a lot of attention recently, emphasizing the significance of clearly defined guidelines for handling viral diseases.

Accurate diagnosis via clinical evaluation and laboratory testing is the first step in treating viral infections. For example, molecular assays and fast antigen testing help verify the existence of the influenza virus. As soon as the infection is identified, the affected person must be quickly isolated to stop the spread of the infection.

Simultaneously, supportive care interventions are implemented to improve recovery and ease discomfort, such as maintaining proper hydration and managing symptoms.

Moreover, antiviral medication is essential in the fight against several viral infections. Drugs like zanamivir and oseltamivir are prescribed for influenza to prevent viral replication and shorten the illness's duration. The best outcomes are obtained when antiviral medications are taken within 48 hours of the onset of symptoms, underscoring the significance of prompt intervention. Antiviral prophylaxis may also be advised in cases of severe influenza or high-risk patients to avoid complications and subsequent infections.

Vaccination is critical in preventing viral infections when combined with treatment measures. Vaccines induce the immune system to generate antibodies that defend against particular pathogens. Seasonal strains that are most prevalent are the focus of annual influenza vaccine campaigns, which operate as a preventative intervention to lessen sickness severity and transmission. Furthermore, new approaches like mRNA vaccines, which have shown remarkably effective against emerging viral threats, have been made possible by breakthroughs in vaccine technology.

In order to cure individual patients and stop the spread of viral diseases on a broader scale, public health activities are essential. Surveillance systems track viral activity, making identifying epidemics early and launching focused therapies possible. Travel bans, community-based initiatives, and quarantine policies are used to stop the spread of viruses and protect public health. Public awareness campaigns also encourage a group effort to stop the transmission of viruses by educating the public about preventive measures like mask use, hand hygiene, and social distancing.

Detailed processes are essential to respond to emerging viral threats like coronaviruses effectively. The cornerstone of containment efforts is early discovery through broad testing, contact tracking, and isolation techniques. To achieve population-level immunity and stop further outbreaks, vaccinations that are specifically designed to target particular virus strains must be developed and distributed. Researchers, medical professionals, and legislators must work together to improve procedures and modify action plans in response to changing viral dynamics.

To sum up, detailed procedures for managing certain viral infections involve a multifaceted strategy that includes public health measures, treatment, prevention, and diagnostics. It is imperative to customize therapies to specific viruses' distinct attributes to reduce the impact of viral infections on individuals and communities. Healthcare systems may effectively combat viral threats and protect public health in an ever-evolving landscape of infectious illnesses by following established norms and embracing innovation.

## Long-term strategies for immune support and prevention

Among other things, strengthening the immune system is essential for general health and illness prevention. Although our immune system can repel intruders, it needs ongoing care and support to perform at its best in the long run. Encouraging general vitality and lowering the risk of infections and chronic illnesses can be achieved through sustainable techniques that strengthen the immune system. A comprehensive strategy for immune support includes a range of lifestyle factors, food selections, exercise, stress reduction, and enough sleep.

A healthy, well-balanced diet is one of the critical foundations of immunological function. Antioxidants, phytonutrients, whole grains, lean proteins, and various fruits and vegetables all provide essential vitamins, minerals, and other nutrients necessary for immune system function. Including foods high in zinc, probiotics, vitamin C, and vitamin D can help strengthen immunity. Reducing use of processed foods, alcohol, and refined sugar can also help to improve immunity and reduce inflammation.

Another essential element of long-term immunological support is regular physical activity. In addition to improving cardiovascular health, moderate-intensity exercise, such as brisk walking, cycling, or swimming, also boosts immunity. Exercise increases circulation, which improves immune cell movement throughout the body and strengthens the body's defenses against infections. Furthermore, regular exercise strengthens the immune system by lowering inflammation and enhancing stress management.

Over time, effective stress management strategies are essential for maintaining immunological function. Prolonged stress can lower immune function, increasing the body's vulnerability to inflammation and infections. Including stress-relieving activities like yoga, deep breathing techniques, mindfulness meditation, and time spent in nature can help regulate the body's stress response and boost immunological resilience. Making time for enough sleep is equally important since it promotes healthy immune function by allowing the body to recover and heal.

Immune function increasingly depends on maintaining a healthy gut microbiome. A complex ecosystem of bacteria found in the gut is essential for controlling immune responses. Consuming fiber-rich meals, fermented foods, and prebiotics helps to nourish the gut's beneficial bacteria, which in turn supports a balanced microbiome and bolsters the immune system. Furthermore, probiotic supplements and refraining from overusing antibiotics can help to maintain immune system resilience and gut health.

Maintaining a healthy balance between work, personal obligations, and recreational pursuits is crucial for immune system support and general well-being. Social isolation, a lack of leisure activities, or long-term overwork can all exacerbate stress and impair immunity.

Strong social ties, hobbies, and regular rest periods are critical for maintaining mental and emotional well-being and boosting immunological resilience.

In summary, implementing long-term immune support and prevention techniques necessitates a comprehensive strategy considering numerous wellness and lifestyle facets. Prioritizing gut health, exercise, stress reduction, sleep, diet, and work-life balance can help people build robust immune systems to fight illnesses and sustain good health over time. Regularly putting these tactics into practice, people can become more resilient and empowered to live healthier, more active lives.

The significance of immunological health has received much attention lately, particularly in the wake of international health emergencies. The focus on long-term tactics for immune support and prevention is equally important, even while short-term measures like immunizations and cleanliness practices are critical in preventing immediate risks. This section examines several long-term immune system support strategies, including dietary changes, lifestyle adjustments, stress reduction methods, and natural vitamins and herbs.

First and foremost, the foundation of long-term immune support is eating a good, well-balanced diet. Antioxidant-rich foods include fruits, vegetables, whole grains, lean meats, and other essential elements that support a strong immune system. Probiotics and prebiotics also help maintain a healthy gut microbiota, which is directly related to immunological health. People can foster an environment conducive to the health of their immune system by prioritizing whole, unprocessed foods and reducing their intake of sweets and harmful fats.

In addition to nutrition, leading an active lifestyle boosts immunological resilience considerably. Frequent exercise has been demonstrated to improve circulation, lower inflammation, and encourage the creation of immune-stimulating cells, all of which strengthen the immune system. A range of physical activities, such as strength training, flexibility training, and cardiovascular exercise, can optimize long-term immune health. Additionally, keeping a healthy weight through regular exercise lowers the chance of developing long-term illnesses that can impair immune function.

Stress management is critical in addition to diet and exercise for long-term immunological support. Chronic stress can damage the immune system by raising stress hormones like cortisol, which gradually decreases immunological function. Including stress-relieving activities in daily life, such as yoga, meditation, deep breathing techniques, and mindfulness exercises, may help lessen the damaging effects of stress on the immune system. It's also important to make sure you get adequate sleep, as not getting enough sleep might impair your immunity and increase your susceptibility to illness.

In addition, taking supplements containing organic immune-boosting substances helps strengthen immune function and promotes a healthy lifestyle. Among the most researched supplements for immune support are zinc, echinacea, vitamin C, and vitamin D. These supplements may shorten the duration and severity of colds and other respiratory infections, according to studies. Before starting any new supplement regimen, it is imperative to see a healthcare expert, as each person's needs and health circumstances are unique.

To sum up, developing a holistic approach to health that includes supplementation, exercise, stress reduction, and nutrition is essential for long-term immune support and prevention. Long-term immune system strengthening and disease prevention can be achieved by emphasizing a balanced diet, frequent exercise, stress management practices, and tailored supplements. A current investment in immunological health also represents a future investment in resilience and general well-being.

## Tips for creating personalized herbal protocols

Creating customized herbal regimens requires a systematic and deliberate approach to using botanical remedies' therapeutic potential for specific health objectives and issues. The growing popularity of complementary and alternative therapies that focus on natural and holistic approaches to well-being has led to an increase in the use of herbal medicine. However, Effective herbal protocols must consider several essential variables, including the client's particular needs, medical history, and constitution. This section examines essential advice experts, and amateurs can use to create customized herbal regimens that maximize effectiveness and safety.

Performing a comprehensive client assessment is the first step toward creating customized herbal treatments. The client's medical history, including any allergies, chronic diseases, and current medications, should be thoroughly reviewed for this examination. In addition, learning about the client's dietary preferences, stress management techniques, and environmental exposures can help reveal important details about their general health and potential imbalances. Practitioners can determine the underlying causes of health problems and customize herbal therapies using a holistic assessment approach.

Effective protocols must be created by carefully choosing herbs based on the assessment results and the unique needs of the client, as well as the herbs' medicinal qualities. Herbs have different therapeutic effects; they can be nervine, adaptogenic, immune-stimulating, or anti-inflammatory. Practitioners can identify imbalances and assist the body's natural healing processes by matching the qualities of herbs to the symptoms and constitution of each individual. The selection of herbs with established efficacy and safety profiles for each case is guided by traditional knowledge, scientific research, and clinical experience.

Furthermore, it is essential to consider possible herb-drug interactions and the synergistic effects of herbs to guarantee the security and effectiveness of customized herbal regimens. Certain herbs have the potential to either increase or decrease the effects of specific prescriptions, while others may increase the risk of adverse responses when taken with particular drugs. As a result, practitioners need to be aware of possible interactions and contraindications and, where needed, work closely with clients' healthcare providers.

Furthermore, consumers are better equipped to take herbal therapies safely and successfully when they are informed about the correct dosage, administration, and side effects.

Creating customized herbal blends based on the client's needs can help improve compliance and therapeutic effects in addition to using individual herbs. Combining different herbs with complementary properties and synergistic effects can increase the advantages of the mixture and treat many areas of a client's health issues. Whether formulating teas, tinctures, pills, or topical remedies, practitioners can adapt their creations to their client's tastes, lifestyles, and preferences. Practitioners can produce well-balanced and flavorful blends that facilitate long-term adherence to herbal treatments by combining herbs with varying effects and flavors.

Moreover, combining food and lifestyle advice with herbal remedies can improve overall health results and address underlying imbalances that lead to health problems. The best results from herbal treatments come from supportive lifestyle adjustments like exercise, diet, stress management, and good sleep hygiene. Encouraging customers to develop health-conscious behaviors that complement their unique needs and objectives can increase the effectiveness of herbal remedies and advance general well-being.

To sum up, developing customized herbal regimens necessitates a multimodal strategy incorporating comprehensive evaluation, cautious herb selection, thought for herb-drug interactions, custom mix creation, and holistic lifestyle advice. By customizing herbal therapies to meet the unique needs and health goals of each client, herbalists can optimize therapeutic outcomes and empower consumers to take a proactive approach in their own health and well-being. Herbalism provides a comprehensive framework for fostering vitality and resilience across a range of people by combining traditional wisdom, scientific understanding, and individualized care.

Developing individualized herbal regimens requires a careful and deliberate process that considers several variables, including a person's goals, lifestyle, preferences, and past and present health. This section examines essential strategies for creating personalized herbal protocols that meet each person's specific requirements, stressing the value of working in tandem with licensed herbalists or medical specialists.

Firstly, creating a customized herbal treatment requires first performing a thorough evaluation of the patient's health. Information regarding the person's medical history, present symptoms or health issues, dietary preferences, lifestyle choices, and any drugs or supplements they may be taking may all be gathered as part of this examination. Herbalists can customize their advice to match the individual's goals and unique needs by getting a detailed grasp of their health history and unique circumstances.

Next, when designing a customized protocol, it's critical to consider the energetics and activities of herbs. Herbs have various energetic properties that can affect how they affect the body, such as hot, cold, moist, and dry, as well as therapeutic properties that can stimulate, calm, and tonify. Herbalists can formulate remedies that complement a person's constitution and address specific health imbalances or problems by choosing plants with the correct energetics and activities. For instance, people who are overheated and inflammatory can benefit from cooling and anti-inflammatory herbs; people who are low in energy need tonifying and energizing herbs.

Furthermore, creating efficient herbal regimens requires a thorough understanding of herbal compatibility and synergy concepts. Some herbs can strengthen each other's effects and improve therapeutic results when used in concert, while others might have opposing effects or interactions. In order to minimize the possibility of unfavorable reactions or interactions and accomplish the intended therapeutic benefits, herbalists must carefully choose herbs that complement one another. Additionally, when choosing herbs and creating herbal concoctions, it's critical to consider the person's preferences and tolerances. When creating an herbal regimen, practitioners should consider the preferences of some individuals, such as those with allergies or sensitivities to particular herbs or who prefer specific delivery methods (teas, tinctures, or capsules).

Moreover, creating customized herbal regimens can benefit from integrating ancient knowledge with modern research. Modern scientific research offers evidence-based support for the safety and efficacy of herbs, while traditional herbal wisdom offers insightful knowledge about herbs' therapeutic qualities and applications. Herbalists may base their recommendations on scientific facts and conventional wisdom to ensure the safety and efficacy of the herbal therapies they prescribe. Herbalists may enhance their practice and give their customers the best, most evidence-based care by keeping up with the most recent research results and advancements in herbal therapy.

In summary, developing individualized herbal protocols necessitates a thorough comprehension of each patient's condition as well as the energetics, actions, and synergies of many herbs. Herbalists can create customized protocols that meet each individual's specific requirements and objectives by carrying out in-depth examinations, taking into account individual preferences and tolerances, and fusing traditional knowledge with cutting-edge research. For individualized herbal interventions to be effective, safe, and satisfying, herbalists and clients must work together. People can use customized herbal protocols to sustainably and holistically support their health and well-being by utilizing plants' medicinal properties.

# CHAPTER XI

# Resources and References

## Recommended books, websites, and organizations for further learning

The search for knowledge is easier than ever in the digital age. Many resources are available to learn something new, expand your knowledge on a particular topic, or keep up with current events and research. This section promotes ongoing education and personal development by highlighting suggested books, websites, and organizations in various subjects.

Books are ageless archives of information providing viewpoints, knowledge, and experiences gathered over centuries. Classics like Eckhart Tolle's "The Power of Now" and Napoleon Hill's "Think and Grow Rich" offer priceless advice on obtaining prosperity and inner peace for anybody interested in personal development and self-improvement. Books like "The Effective Executive" by Peter Drucker and "Start with Why" by Simon Sinek provide practical tactics for effective leadership and organizational success in professional development. Academic textbooks and scholarly works also offer in-depth coverage and reliable information for anyone looking to broaden their views and delve into particular areas.

Websites have become dynamic portals to many resources and information on various topics. Online courses ranging from computer science and data analysis to literature and philosophy are offered by reputable universities and organizations worldwide through websites such as Coursera, Udemy, and Khan Academy.

With the ease and flexibility these platforms offer, students can quickly pick up new abilities and information. In addition, websites such as Medium and TED lectures provide an abundance of thought-provoking articles, lectures, and presentations on various subjects, making them excellent resources for learners and inspiration.

Besides books and online, several organizations are essential for promoting education and information sharing in particular domains. For those in the fields of psychology and engineering, respectively, professional societies such as the American Psychological Association (APA) and the Institute of Electrical and Electronics Engineers (IEEE) offer publications, resources, and networking opportunities. Similarly, non-profits promoting human rights and global health, including Amnesty International and the World Health Organization (WHO), provide educational resources, campaigns, and volunteer opportunities for those enthusiastic about social causes. People can contribute to worthwhile projects and efforts, meet like-minded professionals, and obtain insightful knowledge by getting involved with these organizations.

Furthermore, the rise of online forums and communities has transformed knowledge exchange and cooperation between people with similar interests and backgrounds. Users can ask questions, share thoughts, and participate in debates on various topics on websites like Reddit, Quora, and Stack Overflow, from science and technology to the arts and culture. Similarly, niche online communities offer venues for cooperation, knowledge sharing, and professional networking within particular fields. These communities include software developer-focused sites like GitHub and researcher-focused sites like ResearchGate. Through active participation in these virtual communities, people can access collective intelligence, gain knowledge from the experiences of others, and remain up to date on the most recent advancements in their area of interest.

In conclusion, people looking to start a lifelong learning and personal development journey will find that suggested books, websites, organizations, and online forums are all beneficial tools. Through examining various information sources and interacting with respectable establishments and virtual communities, people can enhance their understanding, perfect their abilities, and maintain a competitive advantage in a constantly evolving global landscape. Using these tools can improve your life and enable you to realize your full potential, regardless of whether you're a professional, student, or just a naturally interested learner.

Pursuing knowledge has never been more accessible in today's fast-paced world when knowledge is readily available at our fingertips. With so many resources at our disposal, selecting the ones that are trustworthy, comprehensive, and appropriate for our goals and requirements can be difficult.

This section presents a wide range of suggested books, websites, and organizations that cover a variety of subjects and areas to assist readers in embarking on a lifelong learning journey.

Books have always been ageless stores of knowledge, providing deep understanding, fascinating stories, and helpful advice on various topics. Classics like Elizabeth Gilbert's "Big Magic" and Viktor Frankl's "Man's Search for Meaning" encourage readers to find creativity, purpose, and resilience in adversity. They are a great place to start for anyone looking to grow personally and learn about themselves. Similarly, publications like Brené Brown's "Dare to Lead" and Simon Sinek's "Start with Why" offer priceless tactics for encouraging creativity, teamwork, and genuine leadership in the context of professional growth and leadership. Furthermore, academic textbooks and scholarly works provide thorough coverage and rigorous analysis for those who wish to deepen their knowledge of specific topics or disciplines. They are invaluable resources for researchers, students, and lifelong learners alike.

Websites have become dynamic portals to resources, information, and engaging educational opportunities. Online learning environments such as Coursera, Udemy, and Khan Academy provide various courses covering topics from data analytics and computer science to the humanities and social sciences. With the help of these platforms, students can expand their knowledge of complex subjects, gain new skills, and obtain certificates or credentials from prestigious colleges and organizations throughout the globe. Furthermore, websites such as TED Talks and Medium provide a wealth of informative lectures, interesting articles, and captivating multimedia content for those with a curious mind. As such, they are indispensable resources for inspiration and education.

Organizations are essential for promoting creativity, teamwork, and learning in specific disciplines and sectors. Professional societies like the American Psychological Association (APA) and the Institute of Electrical and Electronics Engineers (IEEE) offer publications, networking opportunities, and resources for those working in psychology, engineering, and related subjects. Similarly, non-profits such as the World Economic Forum and UNESCO concentrate on sustainable development and global education, providing policy advocacy, research, and capacity-building programs to solve urgent social issues. People can access state-of-the-art research, network with like-minded professionals, and effect significant change in their communities and beyond by getting involved with these organizations.

Furthermore, the growth of online forums and communities has made information sharing more accessible and enabled people with similar interests and backgrounds to work together. Users can ask questions, share thoughts, and participate in debates on various topics on websites like Reddit, Quora, and Stack Overflow, from science and technology to the arts and culture. Similarly, niche online communities offer venues for cooperation, knowledge sharing, and professional networking within particular fields. These communities include software developer-focused sites like GitHub and researcher-focused sites like ResearchGate. Through active participation in these virtual communities, people can access collective intelligence, gain knowledge from the experiences of others, and remain up to date on the most recent advancements in their area of interest.

In conclusion, those starting a lifelong learning and personal development journey can significantly benefit from the assistance of suggested books, websites, organizations, and online communities. Through various information sources and interactions with respectable institutions and virtual communities, people can expand their knowledge on various topics, learn new abilities, and remain current on advancements in the areas they are interested in. Using these resources can enhance your educational journey and enable you to reach your most significant potential, regardless of whether you're a student, a professional looking to progress your career, or just a curious mind ready to explore the enormous expanse of human knowledge.

## Glossary of herbal terms

Using plants for therapeutic purposes or herbalism involves a vast lexicon of words and phrases. Anyone interested in herbal medicine, whether as a consumer, practitioner, or enthusiast, must understand these concepts. This section aims to offer a thorough dictionary of terms related to herbs, encompassing important ideas, botanical terminology, preparation techniques, and therapeutic principles.

Herbs, known as "adaptogens," support general resilience and equilibrium while also assisting the body in adjusting to stress. Ginseng, Rhodiola, and ashwagandha are a few examples.

Infusion: Plant material is steeped in hot water to extract the active ingredients used to prepare herbal medicines. Herbal teas are typically made with this.

Decoction: To extract therapeutic components, plant material, such as roots, bark, or seeds, are boiled in water. More rigid plant components that need to be heated for a more extended period to release their medicinal compounds are frequently treated with this technique.

Tincture: To extract the active ingredients from plant material, tinctures are concentrated liquid extracts created by soaking the substance in glycerin or alcohol. Tinctures are prized for their strength and extended shelf life.

Herbs are steeped in carrier oil, like coconut or olive oil, to extract their medicinal qualities and create infused oils. These oils can be applied topically for therapeutic, skin care, and massage applications.

Herbalism: The use of plants medicinally, combining holistic concepts, current science, and traditional knowledge to enhance health and well-being, is known as herbalism.

A thorough collection of medical ingredients, such as minerals, plants, and animal products, along with their intended applications, dosages, and therapeutic qualities, is called a materia medica.

The study of plants' chemical makeup and characteristics, such as their active ingredients, bioavailability, and pharmacological effects, is known as phytochemistry.

Herbal actions: These are the medicinal qualities or effects of herbs, such as nervine, analgesic, anti-inflammatory, or diuretic.

Herbal energetics: This theory, based on traditional medical systems, divides herbs into classes depending on their energetic characteristics, such as hot, cold, moist, or dry. These characteristics are thought to affect how they affect the body and aid in restoring equilibrium within.

Blends of several herbs selected for their synergistic effects and customized to treat particular health issues or diseases are known as herbal formulations. Formulating topical treatments, tinctures, teas, or capsules is possible.

Dosage: Usually stated in terms of weight, volume, or concentration, dosage describes the appropriate amount of herbal medication to be applied or taken. A correct dosage is necessary to guarantee both efficacy and safety.

**Herbal contraindications: Owing to possible** interactions, adverse effects, or safety concerns, there are situations or conditions in which particular plants should be avoided. When taking herbal medicine, especially in conjunction with pharmaceuticals or other therapies, it is imperative to take contraindications into account.

Herbal safety: When utilizing herbal medication, herbal safety refers to the procedures and safety measures taken to reduce the possibility of adverse responses or interactions. This entails determining the correct dosage, looking for potentially allergenic substances or poisonous plants, and speaking with licensed medical experts.

Herbal folklore: This is the collection of behaviors, beliefs, and practices that surround the traditional usage of plants for ceremonial, magical, or medicinal purposes. Stories, myths, and customs passed down through the centuries within certain cultures or communities are frequently included in folklore.

Herbal pharmacology is the scientific study of medicinal plants' pharmacological characteristics and modes of action, including how they interact with biological systems, receptors, and pathways.

Herbal monograph: An herbal monograph is an extensive document that offers a wide range of information about a particular herb, such as its pharmacological activities, traditional usage, safety issues, and botanical description.

Herbal certification: For those aspiring to become licensed herbalists or practitioners, herbal certification programs offer instruction, training, and certification. These programs often cover botany, phytochemistry, formulation, materia medica, and clinical practice.

Herbal sustainability: The phrase describes methods and ideologies intended to preserve and ethically gather therapeutic plants to guarantee both their long-term availability and ecological sustainability. This covers ethical sourcing practices, sustainable farming methods, regulations for wildcrafting, and conservation initiatives to save threatened species and their ecosystems.

Herbal advocacy: This refers to the work done to advance policy, research, awareness, and education about herbal medicine. It also includes promoting the use of herbal medicines in healthcare systems and pushing for their improved accessibility, regulation, and integration.

## Index for easy reference

An index offers an ordered list of terms, themes, and references, making it an invaluable tool for navigating complicated texts, books, or databases. Indexes improve the usability and accessibility of the content and enable effective information retrieval in both printed and digital media. This section examines indexes' significance, composition, and how they help readers find specific information efficiently and fast.

Scholarly works, reference books, textbooks, and other publications with a lot of information covering several topics and subtopics must all have indexes. By creating an organized or alphabetical list of terms, concepts, names, and page numbers, indexes allow readers to find pertinent information quickly and easily without reading the entire document in order. Researchers, students, professionals, and enthusiasts who need quick access to specialized information for their work or study may find this especially helpful.

An index's structure usually consists of entries grouped hierarchically or alphabetically. Each entry is accompanied by one or more page numbers or references pointing to the information's specific location inside the document. Single words, phrases, concepts, names of people or organizations, and even cross-references to relevant subjects or subtopics can all be included in entries. Furthermore, to improve readability and clarity for users, indexes may use formatting rules like bold text, italics, or indentation to differentiate between main entries, subentries, and page numbers.

An index does more than just list terms alphabetically; it acts as a navigational aid and guides to help readers navigate and explore the information. Indexes enable readers to swiftly and effectively find particular subjects, concepts, or references by arranging material in an orderly and easily readable manner. Because readers can readily cross-reference several sections or chapters to obtain a comprehensive grasp of the subject matter, this saves time and effort and improves comprehension, retention, and engagement with the information.

In the digital age, indexes have grown to incorporate a range of forms and features to meet the needs of modern readers. Online indexes, search engines, and databases use advanced algorithms, metadata, and keyword indexing to enable quick and accurate information retrieval from sizeable digital content repositories. With a single click or tap, readers may effortlessly move between sections, chapters, or external resources in e-books, websites, and digital periodicals thanks to hyperlinked indexes, which improve the interactive and engaging reading experience.

Indexes are essential for effective information retrieval and navigation in complicated books, documents, and databases. Indexes improve usability, accessibility, and reader engagement by giving users orderly lists of terms, themes, and references to seek specific information quickly and efficiently. Academics, learners, professionals, and enthusiasts who wish to swiftly and readily access, explore, and comprehend a broad range of subjects and topics, whether they be in printed or digital media, will find well-structured indexes to be useful tools.

An index is an essential navigational tool in academic texts, literature, and informational resources. It allows rapid and easy access to specific material in more extensive work. The importance of an index for convenient access is discussed in this section, along with how it can improve the usability, accessibility, and utility of books, documents, and digital content in various fields and disciplines.

An index is a list of keywords, subjects, names, and ideas that are systematically arranged within a text and either accompanied by hyperlinks or page numbers that point readers in the right direction. Through the use of an index, readers can find specific subjects, facts, references, or interesting passages without having to read the full document or book because the information is arranged in a structured and searchable fashion. This helps readers retrieve pertinent material quickly and effectively for research, study, or reference needs, saving them time and effort.

An index is an essential tool in academic works that helps researchers, students, and scholars find relevant material related to their area of study or research interests and traverse complex texts. Authors and publishers can improve their publications' scholarly value and usefulness by making significant terms, concepts, and citations easier to find and retrieve. An index also helps readers better understand the subject matter by allowing them to explore related concepts, track thematic threads, and cross-reference related items.

An index is an essential component that improves the usability and accessibility of non-fiction publications, reference materials, and technical manuals for readers looking for specific information or direction on a given topic. An index helps readers find recipes, places to go, or answers to frequently asked questions quickly, whether in a cookbook, travel guide, or troubleshooting manual. This makes the content more approachable and practical. Similar to this, an index in contracts, legal documents, and regulatory texts aids in the comprehension and interpretation of complicated legal language by assisting stakeholders, policymakers, and attorneys in locating pertinent phrases, sections, or precedents.

Even if they are in a different format, indexes are essential for quick reference in the digital age. Users may now navigate and retrieve information with previously unheard-of speed and precision because of indexing tools like search engines, hyperlinks, and metadata tags. These tools are made possible by the widespread usage of electronic books, online databases, and digital archives. Digital indexes improve user experience and expedite information retrieval by offering extensive search functionality, filtering options, interactive elements, and instantaneous access to particular keywords or phrases.

Additionally, an index helps publishers, editors, and content producers structure and organize their information more efficiently. Authors ensure readers can easily find and understand their work by selecting important terms, themes, and concepts for the index. To guarantee the index's quality, completeness, and relevance to the intended audience, editors also play a critical role in its assessment, optimization, and refinement. A well-designed index improves a publication's general quality and usability and increases its impact and efficacy.

An index is an effective tool for arranging, locating, and obtaining information from books, papers, and digital media. An index helps improve a work's readability, accessibility, and utility by giving readers a road map for navigating its contents. This promotes more effective information retrieval and deeper engagement with the content. Regardless of its format—print or digital—an index is still a crucial part of any extensive reference work, providing readers from a wide range of subjects and domains with access to knowledge and comprehension.

# CONCLUSION

The author has produced a helpful resource, "Unlocking Herbal Antivirals: A Comprehensive Guide to Natural Immune Boosters," which sheds light on the potential of herbal medicines in bolstering the body's defenses against viral infections. The book equips readers with the ability to educate themselves on the wide variety of medicinal plants and effectively utilize their healing capabilities through thorough study and valuable insights.

The writers simplify the field of herbal antivirals by combining traditional knowledge with cutting-edge scientific knowledge, giving users a complete toolkit for healthily boosting immunity. The book emphasizes the value of a holistic approach to well-being and invites readers to include herbal medicines in their daily routines to support resilience and general health.

Furthermore, "Unlocking Herbal Antivirals" highlights nature's vast pharmacy and capacity to counter viral dangers, acting as a ray of hope, particularly during global health emergencies. With its easily understood language and valuable suggestions, the book encourages readers to take control of their health and investigate the abundant advantages of herbal therapy. In summary, this book is a vital resource for anyone looking to harness the potential of herbal antivirals to strengthen their immune system and set out on a path to optimum health.

*Thank you for buying and reading/ listening to our book. If you found this book useful/ helpful please take a few minutes and leave a review on the platform where you purchased our book. Your feedback matters greatly to us.*